How the

BRAIN

Works

About the Cover

The cover is a computer generated, T1-weighted magnetic resonance image of a sagittal plane through the head, acquired using a 3D MPRAGE sequence on a 1.5T Siemens SP MR scanner. It is graciously provided by Dr. Paul Morgan, University of Nottingham, UK.

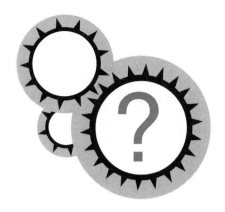

How the
BRAIN
Works

By

MARK Wm. DUBIN, PhD

Professor
Dept. of Molecular, Cellular, and Developmental Biology
University of Colorado
Boulder, CO

Series Editor

LAUREN SOMPAYRAC, PhD

b

**Blackwell
Science**

©2002 by Blackwell Science, Inc.

Editorial Offices:
    Commerce Place, 350 Main Street, Malden, Massachusetts 02148, USA
    Osney Mead, Oxford OX2 0EL, England
    25 John Street, London WC1N 2BS, England
    23 Ainslie Place, Edinburgh EH3 6AJ, Scotland
    54 University Street, Carlton, Victoria 3053, Australia
Other Editorial Offices:
    Blackwell Wissenschafts-Verlag GmbH, Kurfürstendamm 57, 10707 Berlin, Germany
    Blackwell Science KK, MG Kodenmacho Building, 7-10 Kodenmacho Nihombashi, Chuo-ku, Tokyo 104, Japan
    Iowa State University Press, A Blackwell Science Company, 2121 S. State Avenue, Ames, Iowa 50014-8300, USA

Distributors:

The Americas
    Blackwell Publishing
    c/o AIDC
    P.O. Box 20
    50 Winter Sport Lane
    Williston, VT 05495-0020
    (Telephone orders: 800-216-2522; fax orders: 802-864-7626)

Australia
    Blackwell Science Pty, Ltd.
    54 University Street
    Carlton, Victoria 3053
    (Telephone orders: 03-9347-0300;
    fax orders: 03-9349-3016)

Outside The Americas and Australia
    Blackwell Science, Ltd.
    c/o Marston Book Services, Ltd.
    P.O. Box 269
    Abingdon
    Oxon OX14 4YN
    England
    (Telephone orders: 44-01235-465500;
    fax orders: 44-01235-465555)

Acquisitions: Nancy Anastasi Duffy
Development: Nancy Anastasi Duffy
Production: Shawn Girsberger
Manufacturing: Lisa Flanagan
Marketing Manager: Toni Fournier

Illustrations by Mark Dubin
Cover design by Meral Dabcovich, Visual Perspectives
Interior design by Diane Lorenz,
        Lorenz Computer Graphics, Boulder, CO
Typeset by Mark Dubin
Printed and bound by Edwards Brothers, Inc

Permission by the following to reproduce figures is gratefully acknowledged:
    Austin, M.P., Dougall, N., Ross, M. et al (1992b) Single photon emission tomography with 99m Tc-Exametazime in major depression and the pattern of brain activity underlying the psychotic/neurotic continuum. J. Affective disorders 26, 31–44. The relationship to a standard brain atlas is shown in Fig. 1 of Austin et al. (1992b).
    BrainWeb: Simulated Brain Database, <http://www.bic.mni.mcgill.ca/brainweb/>. HTBW pp. 18, 19.
    CTF Systems Inc., <http://www.ctf.com/>. HTBW p. 22-left.
    J. Neurology. Visuo-spatial neglect: a new copying test to assess perceptual parsing. J.C. Marshall and P.W. Halligan. 1993, 240(1): 37-40. p. 38, figures 1b, 3b. © Springer-Verlag. HTBW figure on p. 40-left.
    Trends in cognitive Science. Neuroimaging studies of the cerebellum: language, learning and memory. J.E. Desmond and J.A. Fiez. 1998, 2(9):355-361. p.356, figure 1, with permission from Elsevier Science. HTBW p. 45.
    Professor William Langston, Middle Tennessee State University, <http://www.mtsu.edu/~wlangsto/>. HTBW p. 49.
    Lila R. Dubin. HTBW p. 58-left.
    Michael Lyons, The Noh mask effect: an illusion of facial perception expression, <http://www.mic.atr.co.jp/~mlyons/Noh/noh_mask.html>. HTBW p. 58-right

Printed in the United States of America
01 02 03 04 5 4 3 2 1

Library of Congress Cataloging-in-Publication Data

Dubin, Mark Wm.
  How the brain works / by Mark Wm. Dubin.
    p. ; cm.
  ISBN 0-632-04441-1 (pbk.)
  1. Brain--Popular works.
  [DNLM: 1. Brain--physiology. WL 300 D814h 2001] I. Title.
  QP376 .D788 2001
  612.8'2--dc21
                        2001001882

DEDICATION

This book is dedicated to my lifetime partner and loving wife Alma,

who helps make my life whole,

and

To my teachers and my students, lifetime partners in my learning.

ACKNOWLEDGMENTS

This book would not exist without the encouragement, persuasiveness, and support of my friend Lauren Sompayrac. He convinced me that the complex story of the brain could be presented in an interesting and concise way. He also read and commented on the entire manuscript, certainly improving its readability. He is especially responsible for my learning how to prune unnecessary detail and jargon.

My first graduate student, longtime friend, and colleague Anne Rusoff carefully and thoughtfully read and commented on the entire manuscript in her wonderful perceptive manner. My colleague Paul Levitt made helpful suggestions about writing style. My colleague Lisa Menn carefully read and made suggestions about Lecture 5. The editorial staff at Blackwell Science provided continual encouragement, education, and assistance, and displayed more patience than I thought possible.

CONTENTS

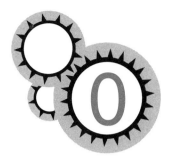

INTRODUCTION

OUTLINE OF THE BOOK

The human brain is the single most complex machine ever constructed. It is the product of a long chain of evolutionary events. Billions of nerve cells, most with thousands of interconnections, are the basis of the unique experience we call humanness. The brain is also the basis of our interactions with the world. Indeed, it is the organ responsible for realizing there is a "me" and there is world that is different from me. This book presents the principles of its functioning.

The book concentrates on the human brain and has the following organizational plan. It starts (Lecture 1, Components) with a presentation of the players—nerve cells—their organization, and their ways of communicating with each other. This lecture and the following one about the techniques used to study the brain (Lecture 2, Exploring) provide a basis for the functional presentations that follow. The logic of Lectures 3 to 5 is to move from a discussion on acquisition of knowledge about the world (Lecture 3, Sensing) to one on the actions that are responses to that knowledge, namely, movement (Lecture 4, Acting) and language (Lecture 5, Communicating). Then, we have a basis for studying the internal realities that intervene between sensation and action, namely, emotions (Lecture 6, Feeling) and awareness and intent (Lecture 7, Thinking). The book then addresses how we organize all of these activities through learning and remembering, including aspects of basic brain development (Lecture 8, Changing). It culminates in a discussion of how "the brain is the organ of the mind" and what we know about consciousness (Lecture 9, Being).

HOW TO USE THIS BOOK

These lectures are purposely concise and colloquial so that you can read them quickly and easily, getting an overall view of the subject. Each lecture can be read on its own in one sitting, in any order. The book is not intended to be a dictionary of terms or to replace other, truly complete presentations about the nervous system. Rather, I hope it provides a clear understanding of principles and basic structure so you can embellish this knowledge with important and interesting details presented in other books and lectures. For those whose recall of the fundamentals of the nervous system is a bit murky, the first two lectures might be useful to read first. Be careful in your reading not to confuse my descriptions with explanations. For example, explaining in detail how photoreceptors in the retina function at molecular and cellular levels would be the subject of a book all by itself. Here, it is described in a few sentences.

Three types of reviews are built into the text. Each lecture opens with a brief review of key concepts presented in the previous lecture. As well, each lecture contains material printed in blue, indicating important ideas. Thus, you can review a lecture by just reading the blue text and examining the figures. Finally, terms defined in italics are summarized in the glossary.

You are invited to visit the Internet site that I maintain in association with this book. The book is intentionally devoid of references, consistent with the "colloquial voice" that is intended in the "How It Works" series. The Web site is meant to address this omission. It has links to resources and references related to the topics presented here, organized by lecture. The URL is <http://dubinweb.com/brain/>.

COMPONENTS

The human brain contains about 100 billion nerve cells and several times that many supporting cells called *glial cells*. Each *neuron* communicates with many others, together giving rise to the overwhelming richness and complexity of the brain's neural circuits. Understanding the basic cellular biology that underlies this complexity requires learning only a few concepts about the structure and function of typical neurons and their organization. That is the purpose of this lecture.

Terminology note: *Neuron* is the one-word synonym for "nerve cell." It is used to avoid confusion with the term *nerve*, the name for a bundle of axons such as the optic nerve.

BRAIN CELL STRUCTURE

A neuron is a cell much like any other. Its cell body (synonym: *soma*) contains the usual components including a nucleus, ribosomes, Golgi apparatus, and the like. However, the neuron (*below*) is specialized for rapid communication with other neurons and has unique anatomic components to accomplish that task. A number of protrusions similar to the branches of a tree, called *dendrites*, extend from the soma. These make up the region where the neuron gets its input. A long extension called the *axon* extends from the soma to an output region. There it ends in axon terminals that make contacts, called *synapses*, with other neurons.

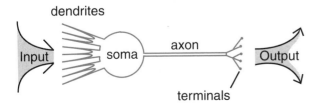

INPUT MAPS

The dendritic regions of neurons come in a wonderful profusion of shapes. To appreciate why this diversity is important, we need to understand another basic principle of brain organization, using a visual system example.

Dealing with visual images is the function of a brain region called the *primary visual cortex* (V1). If you monitor the activity of any V1 neuron, you will find that it responds to visual images only in a very small region in physical space called its *receptive field*. If you monitor a neighboring neuron, its receptive field is adjacent in physical space to that of the first cell. This pattern is true for all cells in the primary visual cortex. You can see that the continuation of the relationship from neighbor to neighbor produces an organized map of the physical world, called a *retinotopic map*.

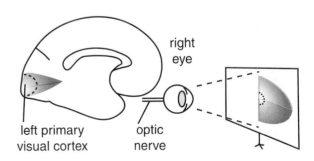

Here, the right eye is looking at an image on a screen. A view of the inside surface of the brain's left hemisphere shows how the image is organized into regularly mapped receptive fields in the primary visual cortex. Note that the region of best vision (the *fovea*) in the center of the visual field (*dashed half-circle*) occupies a disproportionately large part of the map, demonstrating the fact that the map is more than a simple linear projection of the outside world. Instead, more important parts of the input receive more attention because more neurons are available to deal with them.

Cells that respond to adjacent stimuli must interact with one another in the process of analyzing the visual image. The existence of retinotopic mapping makes such functional interaction easy to accomplish because the neurons that "see" adjacent parts of an image are physically near each other in the visual cortex. Similar maps exist for all of the senses, as discussed in Lecture 3.

DENDRITES

Dendrites are not random in size and shape. Instead, the extent of a neuron's dendritic tree and where it is located determines which parts of the map can influence it, thus helping to determine the cell's function. Look (*below*) at this famous example of a type of neuron in the cerebellum called a *Purkinje cell*. On the left, the neuron's dendritic tree is seen face on. Unexpectedly, it is very flat when viewed from the side (*right*). This flatness restricts its access to particular subsets of axonal inputs. The Purkinje cell also demonstrates another feature of many neurons, *spines*, specialized synaptic contact points on the dendrites of cortical cells.

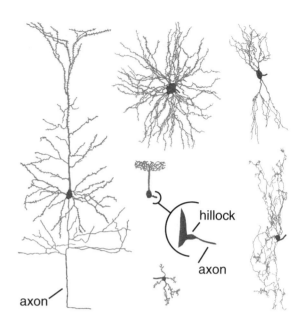

These examples of dendritic trees (*at roughly equal magnification*) show how much they can vary in different brain areas. One interesting difference involves the place on a neuron where the axon begins. Typically, it originates from the soma at an anatomically specialized point named the *axon hillock* (*inset*). However, in some neurons, such as the pyramidal cell (*at left*), the axon originates from one of the dendrites.

AXON TERMINALS

As shown in the next picture, axons usually branch at their end into tens to thousands of small, button-shaped terminals called *boutons*. (*Bouton* is French for "button.") At synapses, these boutons make contact with the dendrites of up to 1000 different neurons, usually making numerous synapses with each. It matters where the synapses are on the dendrites. Boutons that contact a dendrite at its far tip usually have less influence than do ones that synapse near the soma.

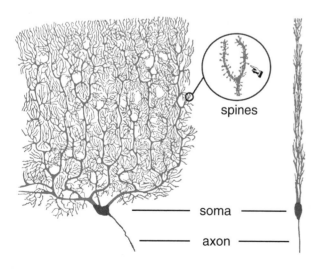

Note: For the Purkinje cell and the next three figures, the soma and the start of each cell's axon are shown in gray to help identify them.

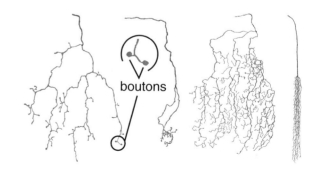

Neurons that carry information from one region of the brain to another can have axons that are quite long. An example is an output neuron with its soma in the brain and an axon that synapses with a neuron at the base of the spine. Some neurons have an axon that splits into a few branches that can end in entirely different parts of the brain. Other neurons communicate only with nearby neurons. Such short-axon neurons are termed *interneurons*. The size of the dendritic tree and of the axonal terminal region is comparable in long-axon and short-axon neurons; all that varies is the length of the axon.

BRAIN CELL FUNCTION

RESTING POTENTIAL

Neurons use an electrical signal called an *action potential* to transmit their message. To understand why and how transmission occurs, it is first necessary to understand the *resting potential*. The potential inside a typical mammalian neuron at rest is about –75 mV (millivolts) relative to the potential in the extracellular space.

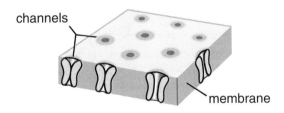

Ions can only cross the neuron's membrane through ion channels that extend from one side of the membrane to the other. A typical patch of neuronal membrane has a few thousand channels per square micron. Each channel is built from protein subunits that form a barrel-like structure with a narrow pore down the center. The channel can be closed or open depending on changes in the shape of the proteins. When open, it becomes a path through which ions can pass from one side of the membrane to the other. Interestingly, these voltage-sensitive pores do not leak; they are either open or closed. Any one type of channel only allows Na^+, K^+, Cl^-, or Ca^{2+} to pass through it. This

selectivity is due to its specific molecular structure. As we will see, the kinds of channels in the membrane vary in different parts of a neuron.

The membrane is permeable to K^+ and barely permeable to other ions when it is at the resting potential because there are many open K^+ channels. The technical way of saying this is that the membrane is *semipermeable*.

K^+ is concentrated and Na^+ is depleted inside the neuron at rest, relative to the extracellular space. These concentration differences are not due to some passive diffusion process; it takes the energy of adenosine triphosphate (ATP) to generate them. To understand how, we need to learn about a molecule called the *Na^+/ K^+ ATPase*. It is a protein "pump" embedded in the neuronal membrane that is fueled by ATP. For each ATP molecule that it splits, the ATPase transports three Na^+ ions from inside the neuron to the extracellular space and two K^+ ions from the extracellular space into the neuron.

What does this pumping have to do with setting up the resting potential? K^+ channels in the soma are open. Thus, because K^+ is more concentrated inside the neuron than outside, K^+ will tend to move out of the neuron via these open channels. Another way this is usually said is that K^+ ions flow down a K^+ *concentration gradient* across the neuron's membrane. The gradient is depicted by the large blue arrow in this figure, pointing in the direction of K^+ movement.

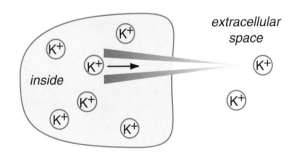

If the concentration gradient was all that mattered, K^+ ions would continue to flow out until the K^+ concentration on the inside and outside was equal. This continued outflow does not happen because an opposing *voltage gradient* is set up as the K^+ leaves. As each positively charged K^+ ion exits the neuron, the inside becomes progressively more negative due to the remaining negatively charged ions. The increasingly negative voltage attracts the positively charged K^+ ions that are inside the cell, making it harder for them to move out down their concentration gradient. The jagged blue arrow that is added in this diagram represents the voltage gradient, indicated by the plus (+) and minus (–) symbols.

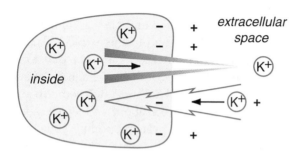

When the voltage inside the neuron reaches –75 mV, the negativity so strongly attracts the positive K^+ ions that the attraction totally offsets their tendency to flow out down their concentration gradient. That is, at the resting potential, equilibrium is reached between the opposing voltage and concentration forces. Additionally, the rate of the Na^+/K^+ pump is voltage-regulated and it almost stops at the resting potential.

This description is a simplification that does not take account of low resting permeability for other ions. In fact, such details are the reason why the resting potential varies among different types of neurons from about –80 mV to –55 mV. All of these details are more fully characterized by electrochemical equations named the Nernst equation and the Goldman equation.

ACTION POTENTIAL

The *action potential* is a voltage change that travels down the axon from the soma to the axon terminals. By way of introduction, here is a brief description of what happens. Depolarization in the dendrites is caused by synaptic input. The positive voltage spreads to the soma, where it causes a voltage change, the action potential, to arise at the axon hillock. The action potential then moves down the axon to its terminals.

The inside of the soma and axon is at the resting potential of –75 mV in the absence of synaptic activation. Special types of voltage-sensitive K^+ channels (*blue*) and Na^+ channels (*black*) in the axon are depicted

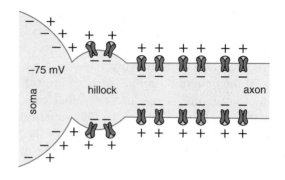

(*above*) in their closed state. These specialized channels are absent in the soma. This graph of voltage versus time is recorded inside the hillock. It initially shows the –75 mV resting potential (*blue*).

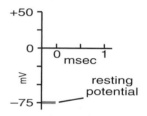

The result of input at excitatory synapses is a change in the resting potential toward 0 mV (called *depolarization*) inside the dendrites of the receiving cell. The depolarization spreads toward the soma and causes its membrane to also depolarize and become less negative. The change is depicted in the next picture by plus signs inside the soma. The depolarization in turn causes a current flow (*indicated by the arrows*) from the soma into the more negatively charged axon hillock. This current starts to depolarize the hillock.

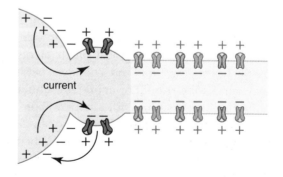

As mentioned, the Na^+ channels in the axon have the property of being voltage-sensitive. Because of this property, when the invading current depolarizes them, it causes a change in channel shape that opens the pore. The open channel lets Na⁺ ions, which are more concentrated outside the neuron, flow down their concentration gradient into the axon.

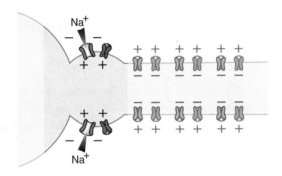

The inward movement of positive charge further depolarizes the axon. If the initial current at the hillock is strong enough to open enough Na⁺ channels, it causes the voltage inside the axon to quickly depolarize even more, and reach a *threshold* value (*left voltage trace below*). At that point all of the hillock's voltage-sensitive Na⁺ channels open, letting more Na⁺ enter. The rapid flow continues until a transmembrane potential of about +20 mV is reached (*right trace*). Then, the drastic voltage change from negative to positive across the membrane causes the Na⁺ channels to close, stopping the Na⁺ ion flow.

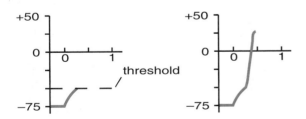

The next thing to be explained is how the voltage change moves down the axon. Notice what happened to the axonal region inside the hillock during the inflow of positive sodium ions; it became very positive. This voltage change sets up a current flow from the hillock to the region next to it, a little farther down the axon. The current then depolarizes that adjacent region and causes the whole cycle to repeat there. That in turn causes a current flow that activates the axon membrane

a bit farther down, and the depolarization moves from region to region all the way down the axon.

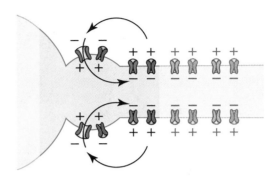

A common analogy is a long trail of gunpowder laid out on the ground. If you use a match to light it at one end, the heat of the burning powder ignites the fresh bit next to it, and that ignites the bit next to it, and so on until the flame travels down the entire string of gunpowder.

Of course, the burned powder cannot ignite again. The axon, in contrast, resets itself to be able to transmit another action potential. As shown in the next figure, resetting happens because the axon membrane contains voltage-sensitive K⁺ channels. These open when the membrane voltage approaches +20 mV at the peak of the action potential, as depicted here.

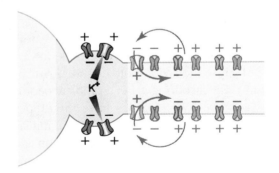

The sudden, large increase in K⁺ permeability allows some of the K⁺ ions inside the axon to quickly flow out down their concentration gradient. As the positive charge leaves the axon, the inside becomes negative again. When it reaches the –75 mV resting potential, the voltage-sensitive K⁺ channels close and that patch of axon is back to its initial state, ready to transmit another action potential. The entire cycle takes about a millisecond (one one-thousandth of a second, abbreviated msec), as shown in this updated graph.

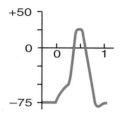

Terminology note: An action potential looks like a transient, spike-like change in voltage when it is recorded with a typical apparatus. Thus, the common synonym for action potential is *spike*, and the frequency of action potentials fired by a neuron is reported as spikes per second.

How are the Na^+ and K^+ concentration gradients restored so that another action potential can be fired? Does the axon need to wait until the Na^+/K^+ pumps rebuild the gradients? It does not, because less than one in 100,000 ions actually crosses the membrane during an action potential. Thus, one action potential does not significantly change the ionic concentrations that are the basis of the resting potential. Although the Na^+/K^+ pumps are not needed to immediately reset the axon, they do work to restore appropriate resting concentrations over the long run as thousands of action potentials occur.

When the action potential is part way down the axon, why doesn't current spread back toward the soma and cause the action potential to move back up the axon? Such backfiring is not a problem because the voltage-sensitive Na^+ channels have the property of being refractory; it takes a few tenths of a millisecond for them to recover their initial configuration. Current that is flowing back up the axon during that time cannot cause them to open, and leaks away before they are reset. Thus, a patch of axon cannot fire another action potential for about 0.5 millisecond due to the refractory Na^+ channels, giving rise to the name *refractory period* for the pause.

It is important to recognize that the action potential remains constant in size as it continuously regenerates itself and moves down the axon. In fact, you should realize that the process that generates the action potential guarantees that all the action potentials in the axon are the same size. Therefore, a neuron cannot change how strongly it signals to other neurons by firing larger or smaller action potentials. Instead, it does so by firing at a different spikes per second rate. Signal strength is indicated by changes in action potential rate, not size.

Interlude—*Episodic Ataxia*

At age 14 George started having brief episodes of loss of muscular coordination (called *ataxia*) and loss of balance. Over the years the length of these episodes increased and by age 40 they lasted for days and were more severe. During an attack he is unable to walk, has slurred speech, and loses control of his extremities. Many of his relatives have the same disease, a rare hereditary condition called *episodic ataxia* (EA). Now that you know about the role of ion channels in the axon, you can understand the basis of EA.

There are many different types of voltage-sensitive K^+ channels. Each is constructed from slightly different protein subunits and has slightly different properties, such as how long the pore takes to open and close. Any one type of neuron usually has only one kind of K^+ channel in its axon, giving its action potential a characteristic width from start to finish. The temporal width is usually in the range of 0.5 to 1.0 millisecond and determines how long the axon terminals signal to their target dendrites. Different neural circuits use this property to fine-tune their activity.

In individuals with EA there is a dominant mutation in one of the genes that codes for the protein designated Kv1.1. The mutation causes the action potentials in the axons that have these channels to have an abnormal width. Researchers are still trying to understand how this abnormality disrupts the functioning of the pathways involved, and why the attacks are episodic rather than continuous. Knowing that a mutated K^+ channel is at the heart of the problem will guide these studies and may eventually lead to the design of helpful drugs.

Given that there are a few-dozen different channel types in the Na^+, K^+, Ca^{2+}, and Cl^- families, it is not surprising that other inherited conditions are being discovered to be axon conduction diseases called *channelopathies*.

MYELIN

Most axons are wrapped in an insulating sheath so that they can conduct action potentials very quickly. Speeds of propagation of 50 m/sec are common. Action potential conduction speed is related to axon diameter because thicker axons have lower electrical resistance. For certain axon classes, speed is not particularly important and being thin and slow is not a problem. Such axons have no sheath. However, an anatomic specialization called the *myelin sheath* is needed to achieve the higher speeds required in most axons. The sheath is made of layers of myelin built up from the membrane of glial cells that wrap around the axon.

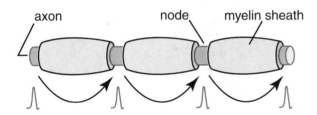

The myelin sheath is a physical and electrical insulator that keeps current from easily entering or leaving the axon. At regular intervals of about a millimeter, there are *nodes* where there is no myelin wrap. These nodes are the only places on the axon where voltage-gated channels are found and where ionic current can flow. Thus, when an action potential occurs at a node, its resulting current flow cannot easily leak out where the myelin-wrapped segments occur, and instead it quickly depolarizes the next node, thus saving conduction time. The action potential occurs at but not in between the nodes, jumping quickly from node to node in a process called *saltatory conduction*. Nodes cannot be too far apart, however, because there is a small amount of ionic leakage in the sheathed regions.

NEURONAL INTERACTIONS

Neurons communicate with each other using neurochemicals called *synaptic transmitters*. These substances are released at specialized contacts called *synapses*. (The word *synapse* comes from a Greek root that means "to clasp.") Like two hands that clasp, the two neurons that interact at a synapse are in very close contact, and just like the two hands, they are not physically continuous. Thus, a way is needed to get the message from the *presynaptic* (sending) side, across the narrow gap to the *postsynaptic* (receiving) side.

SYNAPSE ANATOMY

The physical structure of a synapse suggests how it functions. It is too small to be resolved with a light microscope. Instead, an electron microscope is used to visualize very thin cross sections cut through the synaptic region. The extreme thinness gives a two-dimensional view such as in this actual electron micrograph (in which all surrounding cellular tissue is whited out to emphasize the synapse).

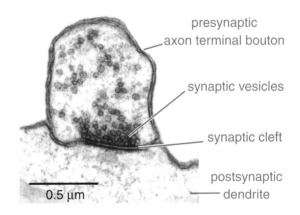

The scale bar shows 0.5 μm (1 μm equals one one-millionth of a meter). To get a sense of how small this size is, realize that the period at the end of this sentence is about 500 μm in diameter. A cross section through one bouton is shown. Only a small part of the postsynaptic dendrite is visible. The segment of the axon that leads to the terminal bouton is not seen because it is not in the plane of this thin cross section.

Every one of an axon's terminal boutons forms the presynaptic side of one synapse. The postsynaptic side is the dendrite (or dendritic spine) of a receiving neuron. The region where the two cells are in closest contact consists of membranes that contain specialized proteins involved in the synapse's function. The space between the presynaptic and postsynaptic side is named the *synaptic cleft*. A prominent identifying feature of a synapse is the cluster of tiny membranous bags called *synaptic vesicles* near the cleft on the presynaptic side. These vesicles contain neurotransmitter molecules.

SYNAPSE PHYSIOLOGY

A series of adjacent thin sections is photographed and then used to build a diagrammatic model to visualize the entire structure of one synapse. Often, a "cartoon," such as this one, is then reconstructed to emphasize the important components and their function.

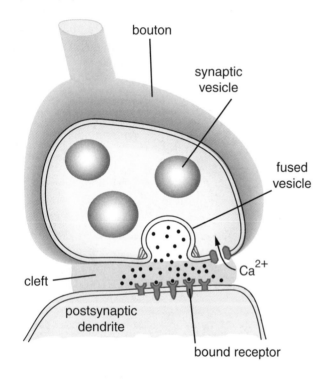

The major anatomic and functional features of this bouton shown in the midst of activation are as follows:

• Contact between the bouton and the dendrite is maintained by a mesh of structural molecules in the cleft (*gray shading*) that holds the two sides together.

• When the action potential reaches the bouton, it causes the interior to depolarize. The depolarization in turn causes voltage-sensitive Ca^{2+} channels that are embedded in the presynaptic membrane to open. Ca^{2+} rushes in because it is at a higher concentration outside the bouton than inside.

• The entering Ca^{2+} causes interaction between specialized protein molecules (*thin gray lines*) bound on

the outside of the vesicle and on the inside of the presynaptic membrane. This causes fusion of the vesicle with the presynaptic membrane, its opening, and the release of its contents to the extracellular space of the cleft. (Excess membrane is reabsorbed later, at the edge of the synapse.)

• Neurotransmitter molecules (*black dots*) that were in the vesicle diffuse across the cleft and bind to receptor molecules embedded in the membrane of the dendrite on the postsynaptic side.

• Receptors to which transmitter molecules bind change their shape and initiate events inside the postsynaptic dendrite.

The entire sequence is terminated in about a millisecond to allow the next signal to arrive. Termination is accomplished by removal of the transmitter molecules from the cleft. For some transmitter substances, such as acetylcholine, this occurs when they are broken down into inactive components by an enzyme permanently present in the cleft. For others, such as serotonin, a pump-type molecule in the presynaptic membrane transports the transmitter molecules back into the bouton where they are reused after repackaging into new vesicles. Still other transmitters, such as the peptide modulators, diffuse away into the surrounding extracellular space and are degraded by nonspecific enzymes.

ACTIVATION AND INHIBITION

The postsynaptic dendrite can be excited or inhibited depending on the nature of the neurotransmitter and the postsynaptic receptor. Excitation occurs when the postsynaptic receptor that binds a neurotransmitter molecule is a Na^+ channel that is normally closed in the unbound state. For example, the binding of the excitatory neurotransmitter glutamate to its receptor causes a pore in the receptor to open and let Na^+ ions enter the dendrite. The influx of Na^+ causes a small depolarization, called an *excitatory postsynaptic potential (EPSP)*. The EPSP causes current to flow from the depolarized region toward the axon hillock. As shown here, a typical EPSP lasts about a millisecond. If

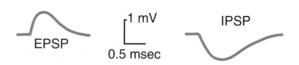

enough dendritic regions are activated simultaneously, their combined EPSP is strong enough to depolarize the hillock to threshold, and an action potential is initiated, carrying the message onward.

Inhibition occurs when an inhibitory transmitter, such as gamma-aminobutyric acid (GABA), binds to its receptor and causes a pore in the receptor to open and let Cl⁻ enter. The flow of Cl⁻ ions makes the inside of the dendrite more negative (a condition called *hyperpolarization*). The resultant voltage change is called an *inhibitory postsynaptic potential* (*IPSP*). It is the opposite of excitation and moves the hillock voltage away from the action potential threshold.

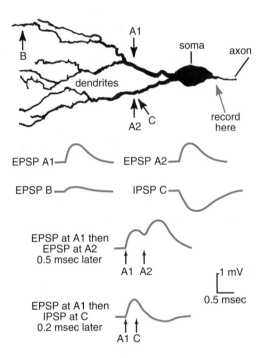

This figure shows a soma and dendrites to illustrate how postsynaptic potentials interact based on where the synapses are on the dendrites. The farther out on a dendrite that a synapse is, the less influence it has on the voltage at the soma (*compare EPSP A1 with EPSP B*). The diminished influence is due to the leakage of synaptic-induced current during its transit over the long distance from the dendrite's end to the axon hillock. EPSPs that occur close together in time are additive (*A1 closely followed by A2*), moving the hillock closer to threshold than either EPSP would alone. The opposite occurs when an IPSP arrives during an EPSP (*A1 followed by C*), cutting short excitation because the two postsynaptic potentials effectively cancel each other out.

In summary, action potentials in the presynaptic cell can cause either excitation, leading to an increase in spike activity, or inhibition, which brings about a decrease of firing in the postsynaptic cell.

SYNAPTIC TYPES AND TRANSMITTERS

So far, we have dealt with what is called *ionotrophic* synaptic transmission, where receptors open pores that allow the direct flow of ions into the dendrite. Not all synaptic receptors are the ionotrophic type. Some are separated from the ion channels that they control and use second messenger–type signaling. For example, when the inhibitory transmitter glycine binds to its receptor, a change in receptor shape causes the activation of a molecule inside the dendrite, called a *G-protein*, which ultimately causes inhibition by the opening of Cl⁻ channels. This multistep process is slower than the direct ionotrophic one and can take many milliseconds to build up to full effect. But that effect, called *metabotrophic*, usually lasts longer than ionotrophic activation. Some postsynaptic cells have both ionotrophic and metabotrophic receptors.

Some neurons simultaneously release both their main transmitter and another one called a *peptide neuromodulator* that makes postsynaptic receptors either more or less responsive to their primary transmitter. In all cases, however, it is important to know that any one neuron releases the same neurotransmitter, or neurotransmitters, at all of its synapses.

Typically, each kind of neurotransmitter in the brain is usually excitatory or inhibitory. However, in some cases, a dendrite can have synaptic receptors that are different from the common ones and lead to inhibition rather than activation, or vice versa.

The figure shows the structure of some major neurotransmitters, to emphasize the point that all are small molecules that can readily diffuse in aqueous environments. Some transmitters are gas molecules, such as nitric oxide (NO) and carbon monoxide (CO), that work by stimulating the activity of second messenger molecules postsynaptically.

Finally, there are synapses that use no transmitter at all. Instead, a special channel bridges the presynaptic and postsynaptic membranes and provides a direct ionic path between them. These *electrical synapses* let current flow from the presynaptic action potential into the postsynaptic dendrite and directly depolarize it.

Neuronal interactions can be very complex because the various types of synaptic activities allow for a remarkably diverse fine-tuning of neuron to neuron communication.

BRAIN CELL ORGANIZATION

Brain cells are grouped into distinct regions that are functionally specialized. These regions are basically the same from person to person, and each usually has specific functions. (Such a collection of related neurons is often called a *nucleus*.) For example, the cells of the lateral geniculate nucleus in the thalamus relay visual signals from the eyes to the rest of the brain. Homologous places in every human's brain usually have identical functions. Many areas have multiple, related functions, and complex functions are carried out in many areas.

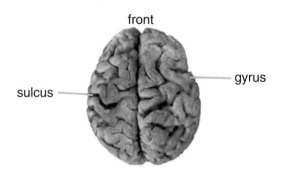

The brain's most obvious feature is the cerebral cortex (synonym: *cerebrum*). It is divided into two

hemispheres, as in the human brain seen here viewed from above. The first structures to note are the mountain-like *gyri* (singular: *gyrus*) and the slits, called *sulci* (singular: *sulcus*), that separate them. All neurons lie within only a few millimeters of the surface of the cortex. Thus, the infolding of gyri increases the surface area of the brain, letting it have more neurons than it would if its cortices were smooth and flat. Highly folded brains are an evolutionary specialization found mainly in primates. Animals lower on the evolutionary scale tend to have smooth cortices.

The hemispheres are not mirror images. The exact patterns of packing of the gyri are similar but not identical. In addition, the left hemisphere is usually a bit larger in humans, especially at the front. This size difference reflects specialized functions located in the left hemisphere, such as language processing, and to a lesser extent, handedness.

TERMINOLOGY

The following diagrams provide a basic vocabulary of anatomic terms. Mastering the entire vocabulary is a daunting task because there are about 800 named structural features in the human brain. Worse, each has about four or five synonyms. This diagram illustrates the common terms for the front, back, top, and bottom of the brain, as well as names for planar sections through it.

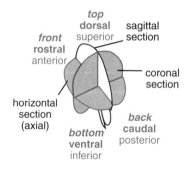

Each hemisphere of the cerebral cortex consists of four lobes (*next figure*) that are defined by the especially deep sulci between them. Probably the most important lobe-related fact is that the frontal lobe is more developed and larger in humans than in any other animal, even our nearest primate relatives. We

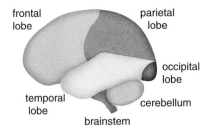

frontal lobe
parietal lobe
occipital lobe
cerebellum
temporal lobe
brainstem

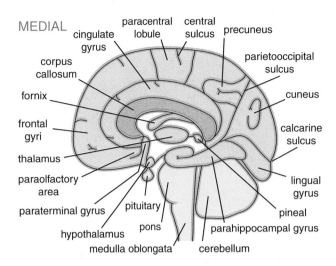

MEDIAL
cingulate gyrus
paracentral lobule
central sulcus
precuneus
corpus callosum
parietooccipital sulcus
fornix
cuneus
frontal gyri
calcarine sulcus
thalamus
lingual gyrus
paraolfactory area
pineal
parahippocampal gyrus
paraterminal gyrus
pituitary
hypothalamus
pons
medulla oblongata
cerebellum

will see in later lectures that it is the basis of many of the higher functions that define us as human.

Connecting the cerebrum to the spinal cord is a specialized region called the *brainstem*. It controls many of the body's basic physiologic functions, such as breathing. Tucked below the cerebrum is the cerebellum. Its most familiar role is in the coordination of movement. However, recent studies have shown that it also has important roles in learning and memory.

white when a real brain is cut in half, owing to the natural color of the white myelin sheath that surrounds each axon. The white coloration of myelin everywhere in the cerebrum is the basis of the common term *white matter* for the bulk of the inner tissue of the brain. In contrast, the thin layer of cells that make up the first few millimeters of the cortical surface usually appears gray in many anatomic preparations. This coloration is the basis of the term *gray matter* that is often used as slang for our thinking apparatus.

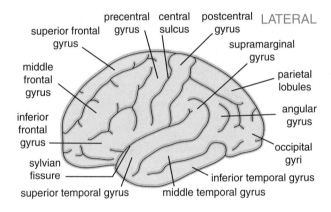

precentral gyrus
central sulcus
postcentral gyrus
LATERAL
superior frontal gyrus
supramarginal gyrus
middle frontal gyrus
parietal lobules
inferior frontal gyrus
angular gyrus
sylvian fissure
occipital gyri
superior temporal gyrus
middle temporal gyrus
inferior temporal gyrus

The figure shows the left hemisphere seen from the outside, with the front at the left, called a *lateral view*. The next figure is a view of the right hemisphere made by cutting the two hemispheres apart down the middle of the brain from front to back and then picturing the exposed surface (called a *medial view*).

Both views show the location of gyri and of a few defining sulci. The medial view also shows a very large region called the *corpus callosum*, which is made up entirely of the axons of neurons that communicate between the two hemispheres. A few gyri and other major brain regions are buried and not visible in these views.

Terminology note: Although the corpus callosum is depicted by a light gray color, it actually looks

Appendix I provides a hierarchical list of important brain regions. It also shows the relationship of commonly used names for brain regions: forebrain, midbrain, hindbrain; and telencephalon, diencephalon, mesencephalon, metencephalon, myelencephalon.

Two other ways to categorize parts of the brain give rise to terms that are commonly used. One method defines regions by the ways their cells are organized in layers and groups (a technique called *cytoarchitectonics*). The anatomist Brodmann used this technique and published a map in 1909 with about 45 different areas defined in the cortex. Therefore, most regions have a "Brodmann area number" that identifies them. A version of his map is in Appendix I. Additionally, many brain regions have an acronym-type name that is related to their function. For example, near the center of the occipital lobe a region defined as Brodmann's area 17 is the first place in the cortex that receives visual input. So, it is also called V1, a shorthand for "Visual 1."

Interlude—*Hydrocephalus*

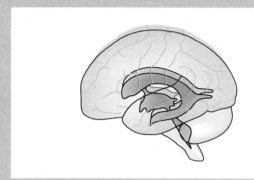

This picture shows the *ventricles* (*blue*), important, nonneuronal structures buried deep within the brain. They are filled with *cerebrospinal fluid* (CSF) that bathes the brain surfaces and provides both a mechanical cushion and a source of ions necessary for neuronal function.

A normal brain contains about 150 mL of CSF that is renewed by special ventricular cells (the *choroid plexus*) about every 6 hours. Continuous production of CSF is needed because of adsorption of CSF by other ventricular cells.

If the normal flow of CSF is blocked during fetal development, or if CSF is grossly over-produced or underabsorbed, a condition known as *hydrocephalus* can occur. When mild, it can be treated postnatally with surgically implanted, artificial tubular shunts that drain the excess CSF. However, when severe, it results in greatly expanded ventricles and a skull almost completely full of CSF. The expansion leaves little room for neurons, and very little brain tissue is present. Such babies usually are stillborn or die soon after birth.

Very rarely, babies with severe hydrocephalus appear neurologically normal at birth and are treated by implanting shunts. These children can grow into normal adults—normal, that is, except for the anatomy of their brains. Brain scans show that their neural tissue is bunched up between the fluid-filled cavity and the skull, with no obvious parts recognizable as gyri or almost any of the other named regions.

What is the point of all the neatly arranged, reproducible brain anatomy if some (rare) folks get along without it? Normally, it helps to ensure the right pathways and connections between the various brain regions. But the existence of a few normal-behaving individuals with severe hydrocephalus shows that the developmental processes that give rise to basic brain connections can sometimes adapt to severely altered anatomy.

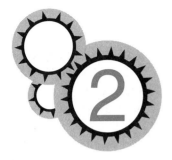

EXPLORING

REVIEW

The first lecture introduced the nuts and bolts of the basic anatomy and function of neurons. Neurons contain all of the typical components of any cell and in addition are specialized to communicate quickly with each other. To accomplish this, a neuron has branch-like dendrites extending from its cell body that are the target of inputs from other neurons at synapses. A single, thin extension—the axon—usually originates at a special point on the cell body and travels to a target region where it branches into a bush-like profusion of individual, button-like terminals (boutons) each of which is part of a synapse onto the dendrite of another neuron. Axons can be very long in order to carry messages from one part of the brain to another, or very short to provide communication with nearby neurons.

A neuron uses changes in voltage to carry signals from region to region within itself, and chemical signaling molecules (neurotransmitters) to convey signals to other neurons. The voltage changes take two forms: the action potential that is actively regenerated as it travels down the axon; and graded postsynaptic potentials (PSPs). These voltage-based signals depend on the fact that the inside of a neuron is at about −85 mV relative to the outside. This resting potential arises from an ATP-powered pump that simultaneously moves sodium out of the neuron and potassium into it, and from a resting permeability to potassium.

Activation at a synapse causes a small voltage change inside the dendrite that makes the dendrite either less negative if it is an excitatory postsynaptic potential (EPSP), or more negative if it is an inhibitory postsynaptic potential (IPSP). Both types of PSPs generate a brief current that flows from the dendrite to the cell body. Normally, many PSPs overlap temporally. If the net result makes the cell body less negative, then voltage-sensitive sodium channels in the initial region of the axon open briefly, allowing sodium to enter and further depolarize the axon. If the summation of PSPs is strong enough, this depolarization reaches a voltage threshold and all of the sodium channels in the initial section of the axon open simultaneously. The inrush of sodium then changes the voltage inside the neuron from negative to about +25 mV. The sodium channels then close spontaneously, and the positivity causes voltage-sensitive potassium channels to open. Finally, as potassium exits the neuron, the voltage returns to the resting potential, causing the voltage-sensitive potassium channels to reclose. This entire action potential sequence lasts about one millisecond. Because of its brief spike-like voltage change, an action potential is usually referred to as a "spike."

The action potential at the initial region of the axon causes current to flow to the adjacent part of the axon, depolarizes that part to threshold, and causes the action potential to regenerate itself in that place. The action potential at this new point of the axon causes current flow to the point immediately next to it further down the axon, generating an action potential there. In this way the action potential "ignites" its way down the axon to the terminal boutons, much like a burning section of a trail of gunpowder ignites the fresh gunpowder next to it.

A key fact about action potentials in a neuron is that each one is the same size as another. Thus, a neuron cannot signal more strongly by firing larger action potentials. Instead, the number of action potentials per second determines the strength of signaling.

When the action potential reaches the end of the axon and causes currents to flow into the terminal boutons, the signal is changed from electrical to chemical. This change is necessary because individual neurons are in close contact, but are not continuous at a synapse. Thus, the high resistance of their outer membranes keeps the action potential from jumping across the synapse. Boutons contain small ball-like inclusions called synaptic vesicles. When the arriving action potential depolarizes a bouton it causes a few vesicles to fuse with the outer membrane of the bouton. They release their content of neurotransmitter molecules into the synaptic region where these small molecules quickly diffuse to the dendritic side of the synapse. There, they bind with specific receptor molecules, leading to the opening of ion channels in the dendritic membrane. The resultant flow of ions is the cause of the PSP. The nature of the neurotransmitter and the receptor molecule's structure and its ionic specificity determine whether the PSP is excitatory or inhibitory.

A typical dendritic tree participates in thousands of synapses. PSPs from those synapses occur with high frequency and thus overlap. The net effect is a continuous variation of the potential at the site of action potential initiation, sometimes reaching threshold and causing an action potential. Thus, every action potential of a particular neuron is the result of the summation of the ongoing activity of inputs from all of the other neurons that contact it at synapses.

Neurons are grouped within the brain in patterns relating to their functions. Local groups of neurons usually have a common function. In a human brain this organization is most grossly reflected in the patterns of gyri and sulci that make up each of the hemispheres of the cerebrum. These infolded regions allow the brain to contain many more neurons than the flat cerebrums of other animals.

It has been possible to record electrical signals from individual neurons inside living brains for about 50 years. This invasive technique cannot be used in people except for rare situations during brain surgery, but its use in animals has led to a basic understanding of brain function. In humans, recording voltage changes at the skull surface, a technique called *electroencephalography* (EEG), has had to suffice even though its interpretation is ambiguous. Some of the ambiguity can be reduced by using the related procedure of recording magnetic fields named *magnetoencephalography* (MEG) at the skull surface, although MEG requires very expensive equipment.

Studies of dead tissue led to most of the detail discussed in Lecture 1. In the twentieth century, the use of x-rays started to provide real images of living brains. However, even techniques such as *computed tomography* (CT) are of limited value because soft tissues such as the brain do not significantly absorb x-rays. The development in the 1980s of magnetic resonance imaging (MRI) as a medical tool changed this limitation; MRI allows soft tissue to be imaged at high resolutions. Recent technical advances in MRI now let us see localized activity in the brain during a particular function, such as the viewing of an object or the thinking of a thought. Similar studies are possible using the research technique called *positron emission tomography* (PET).

How these techniques work is the subject of this lecture. Understanding their use and limitations is important because they are main sources of evidence for the material that makes up the rest of the book.

NEUROANATOMIC IMAGING

TOMOGRAPHY

Many modern brain-imaging methods use the underlying technique of *tomography* (from the Greek root *tomos*, meaning "slice"). It is a concept that is as easy to grasp as slicing an orange.

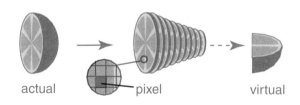

actual   pixel   virtual

The left side of the picture shows a solid half of an orange. To determine what it looks like inside, it must be cut into many adjacent slices. Then, the details of each slice are imaged with the assistance of a computer-based scanner that records the light intensity at each point on the slice. As depicted in the inset, an imaginary grid is superimposed on a slice's image and the average intensity of each square of the grid is determined. Each square is a tiny, local "picture element," giving rise to the shorthand name *pixel*. The more pixels sampled per unit of area, the higher the resolution of the resulting computer representation.

In actual practice, the intensity is not a measure of the surface reflection of the slice. Rather, it is the average of the density of a tiny volume that is made up of the pixel projected from one side of the slice through to the other. Such a "volume element" is called a *voxel*. The computer amasses intensity data for every voxel in every slice. Then, the computer can calculate what any part of the orange would look like from any direction and present that virtual image, such as the piece of the orange shown on page 16.

In sum, tomography is used to generate a three-dimensional model of the brain by imaging adjacent slices which are then reconstructed by software into a solid that can be displayed from any point of view.

COMPUTED TOMOGRAPHY

CT scanning builds up a picture of the brain based on the differential absorption of x-rays. During a CT scan (also called a CAT scan, where the *A* stands for "axial") the subject lies on a table that slides in and out of a hollow, cylindrical apparatus, seen below in cross section. An x-ray source rides on a ring around the inside of the tube, with its beam aimed at the subject's head. After passing through the head, the beam is sampled by one of the many detectors that line the machine's circumference. The beam and detector are narrow, so only a thin slice of the brain is imaged.

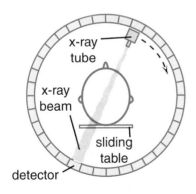

Each detector records the amount of x-ray absorption by an entire pencil-like column of tissue shown by the gray beam in the picture. How is this absorption measure turned into information about individual voxels? Each voxel is part of many columns. This overlap allows the computer to use triangulation-

like techniques to reconstruct the absorption of each voxel in the slice. It is similar to reconstructing the shape of a loaf of bread by shining light at it from three perpendicular directions, recording only the shadows that result, and then using that information to infer the shape of the object casting the shadows.

The table is used to slide the subject down the tube a few millimeters at a time so adjacent slices can be x-rayed in order to image the entire brain. The less the table is moved per slice, the better the resolution. However, such finer movement takes longer and exposes the subject to higher radiation doses.

Images made using x-rays depend on the absorption of the beam by the tissue it passes through. Bone and hard tissue absorb x-rays well. Air and water-filled spaces absorb very little. Soft tissue is somewhere in between. Thus, CT scans reveal the gross features of the brain but do not resolve its structure well. They are good for showing foreign bodies, like bullets and nails, and for detecting tumors and blood clots, which are usually much denser than the surrounding brain tissue.

MAGNETIC RESONANCE IMAGING

MRI works well in soft tissues and gives detailed images of the living brain. It does not expose the subject to harmful x-irradiation. Instead, it uses strong, but safe magnetic fields and radio-frequency (RF) signals. It depends on an atom's property called *spin*. The nucleus of an atom contains positively charged protons and uncharged neutrons. If the number of protons and neutrons is unequal, the nucleus has strong spin. Spin gives it a net magnetic moment, making it somewhat like a tiny bar magnet. Hydrogen is usually imaged in MRI because of its abundance in the body and because its single proton gives it strong spin.

Unlike normal magnets that can be in any orientation, spin comes in only two varieties, spin up and spin down. You can think of spin as tiny magnets, some with their north end pointing up and the others pointing down.

Terminology note: MRI relies on the atom's nucleus and was first called *nuclear magnetic resonance* (NMR) imaging. Patients often equated the word nuclear with unsafe radioactivity, although nothing radioactive is involved. So, NMR got a public-relations face-lift via a new name.

An MRI apparatus is superficially similar to a CT scanner. Again, the subject lies on a table inside a long tube. However, the outer shell is not a detector ring. Instead it is a very powerful magnet with a strength of about 2 teslas (T) or more. (The strength of Earth's magnetic field is 0.6 gauss. One tesla equals 10,000 gauss.) Because the field does not vary, it does not have any harmful magnetic effect on the body. In contrast, oscillating magnetic fields can induce dangerous currents in the brain.

The magnet stays on throughout the MRI scan. Its strong magnetic field aligns most of the atomic nuclei, with their spin pointing in one direction. Then, a transmit-and-receive coil is used to transmit a brief pulse of RF energy at a frequency that is absorbed only by the hydrogen atoms, in a process called *resonance* (hence, that word appearing in the acronym *MRI*). This pulse causes the nuclei to overcome the large, fixed magnetic field and flip their spin to the other direction. It also gives an energy boost that causes all the nuclei to wobble on their axis in exact synchrony. As soon as the RF pulse ends, these nuclei start to return to their pre-pulse condition. The return does not happen all at once. Rather, one nucleus reverts back and then another, the whole process (called *relaxation*) taking a number of milliseconds.

Because the atomic nuclei absorbed energy when the RF pulse made them flip and wobble, they must give up this energy as they relax back to their lower-energy, initial condition. They do so by emitting tiny RF pulses at a characteristic frequency. The relaxation time for two-thirds of the nuclei to flip their spin back is called *T1*. The relaxation time for two-thirds to lose their synchronized wobble is called *T2*. Now the important fact: Because they are due to different kinds of processes, T1 and T2 relaxation times differ in various chemical environments, including in the brain.

The MRI machine can be tuned to specifically measure the time course of either T1 or T2. It does so while very quickly focusing on one small volume (voxel) after another throughout the brain. The entire image takes 2 to 4 seconds to collect.

MRI resolves soft tissues well. Hard tissue, such as bone, usually gives a very weak MRI signal, making it almost transparent. White matter can be distinguished easily from gray matter because of their different water content.

The sagittal section in the next picture, imaged near the midline, shows a typical MRI result. The detail

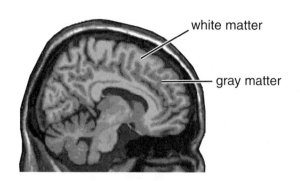

is remarkable, with every sulcus and gyrus being easily recognized. Because of the use of tomographic techniques, any plane, section, or part of the brain can be displayed, such as in the horizontal sections in the next figure that show the differences between T1 and T2 images. The left picture is T1-optimized for white matter; the other picture of the same slice is T2-optimized for gray matter and the fluid-filled ventricles, causing them to appear white.

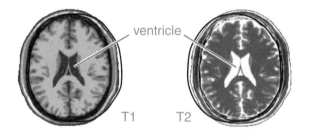

Interlude—*Multiple Sclerosis*

In multiple sclerosis (MS) the myelin sheaths of individual axons are damaged, causing conduction velocity changes that lead to abnormal functioning. The brain regions that are affected vary from patient to patient and in an individual over time. Because of differences from patient to patient, a great variety of apparently unrelated neurologic symptoms can appear in any one person. Thus, diagnosis of early-stage MS is difficult and is now assisted by use of MRI.

The changes in the structure of myelin brought about by MS cause diseased, localized patches of white matter to swell and thus appear fluid-like on MRI scans that are optimized for T2. This horizontal MRI section shows telltale MS

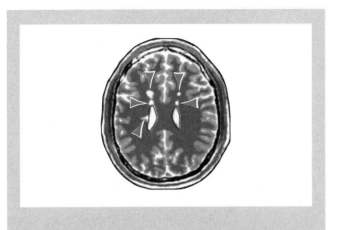

patches (*blue arrows*) that are near ventricles (*white, outlined in blue*).

FUNCTIONAL MAGNETIC RESONANCE IMAGING

Functional MRI (fMRI) detects changes in localized activity in the brain. Its emergence over the past decade is the most exciting recent development in our quest to localize and understand function in the living brain. The technique takes advantage of the fact that a region of the brain that is very active undergoes a local, rapid change in blood oxygen concentration. Because hemoglobin molecules that have bound oxygen have different magnetic properties from unbound ones, the T2 time of the region changes. The effects of the change are detected by first making an MRI image in a passive, control situation and then making one while the task of interest is being performed. When the first image is subtracted from the second, only the active regions with changed oxygen concentrations appear in the image.

For example, in the experiment depicted in this picture, a subject viewed a small visual stimulus presented for many seconds. The blue areas show the averaged T2 activity that occurred in response to the stimulus, superimposed on a T1 image that shows the overall structure of the brain so that areas of interest can be identified. Dark blue indicates a strong response. Not surprisingly, the area activated is in the region of the primary visual (occipital) cortex. It is important to realize that other nearby regions also may have been active but not strongly enough to show up in the fMRI analysis. However, the technique is sensitive enough to allow many of the functional identifications discussed in the following chapters.

Terminology note: This is called the blood oxygen level determination (BOLD) technique. You might reasonably assume that the active region is using up oxygen and that a decrease in blood oxygenation is measured, but the transient dip is too small to detect. However, within about 2 seconds the local capillaries expand and deliver an excess of oxygenated blood. This increase of about 3% over background levels is what fMRI detects. It also can detect significant decreases in regional activity that cause large drops in local circulation.

Images from fMRI experiments are often presented in color. The colors are entirely artificial and are used to make it easier to visualize results. In the figure above, only blue is used, although often a spectral color scale is used, from blue through the colors of the spectrum to red. Blue, a "cold" color, indicates strongly decreased activity, and red, a "hot" color, indicates strongly increased activity. The other spectral colors show gradations between these extremes.

POSITRON EMISSION TOMOGRAPHY

PET and its variant single-photon emission computed tomography (SPECT) use trace amounts of short-lived radioactive isotopes to localize regions where specific molecules of neurobiologic interest are involved in brain function. These techniques make use of the fact that a positron—a "positive electron"—is frequently emitted in radioactive decay events. It travels a tiny distance and meets up with an electron, and then the two annihilate each other, producing two photons that travel in precisely opposite directions. A PET scanner analogous to the scanners we have already discussed detects these photons. A computer triangulates

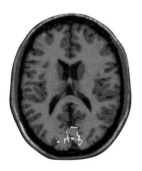

these events to show where in the brain the decay occurred.

One key difference between PET and MRI is that PET can be used to observe a wide range of molecules, whereas MRI is currently limited to looking at hydrogen in water. A tracer molecule of interest such as glucose, or a neurotransmitter, or a molecule that binds to a particular postsynaptic receptor is made radioactive for PET studies using a cyclotron (more commonly called an *atom smasher*). Because the half-life of the radioactive atom (typically hydrogen, carbon, or oxygen) is only minutes, the cyclotron facility and the PET facility must be adjacent, thus limiting PET to a few large, research-oriented medical centers. The quick decay of the tracer's radioactivity allows repeated studies on the same subject. It is important to note that the time needed for the tracer to reach a site of interest in concentration high enough to be detected makes the temporal resolution of PET studies a bit worse than the resolution of fMRI studies.

In SPECT, isotopes that decay with the emission of single photons (usually iodine and technetium) are used. They can be linked as radioactive tracers to molecules without the use of a cyclotron. Therefore SPECT does not require a cyclotron, thus allowing for its use by many more researchers than have access to PET facilities. However, there are two downsides. First, iodine and technetium have half-lives of many hours. The increased duration of radiation to the subject and the long time for the tracer to disappear make repeated observations difficult. Second, only a limited range of biomolecules can have iodine or technetium attached to them and still function. However, with SPECT, the long half-life of the tracers can be used to advantage; a subject injected with the tracer can do some interesting physical task outside of the scanner that could not be done while inside the machine, and then be scanned to localize the tracer molecule.

Interlude—*Alzheimer's or Depression?*

Alzheimer's disease typically develops over many years in old age. The onset of symptoms of forgetfulness and social withdrawal is slow and insidious. There are no good tests to identify it in its early stages. Depression is also a disease that is difficult to diagnose. In elderly persons it is often incorrectly taken to indicate a normal loss of social interest and thus, regrettably, goes untreated. Symptoms of treatable depression resemble early-stage untreatable Alzheimer's.

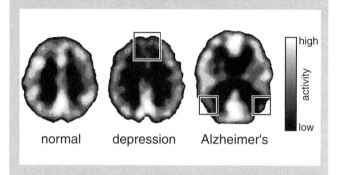

normal   depression   Alzheimer's

Recently, SPECT has begun to offer a way to differentiate between depression and Alzheimer's. The figure shows resting brain activity in normal, depressed, and Alzheimer's-afflicted elderly persons. White indicates high activity and black, no activity, with intensity of gray indicating intermediate levels. The depressed patient shows a characteristic decrease in activity in the frontal regions (*box*) relative to the normal person, while the Alzheimer's patient shows decreased activity in the parieto-temporal regions (*boxes*). Such differentiation avoids misdiagnosis and can indicate the need for treatment for depression.

ELECTROPHYSIOLOGIC TECHNIQUES

MICROELECTRODES

Microelectrodes are used to monitor the firing of individual neurons in response to stimuli. They are long, thin metal probes about a millimeter in diameter for most of their length. They are coated with electrical insulating material except for a region at their tip that is sharpened to a fine point smaller in size than a neuron's soma. The small size allows the tip to be placed next to

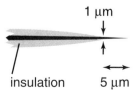

1 μm

insulation   5 μm

the soma where it can record the cell's action potentials. The other end of the microelectrode is connected to electronics that amplify and display the signal.

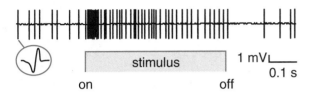

This figure shows a typical result. The time scale is chosen to show the overall response of the cell to the stimulus, ignoring the identical shape of each action potential (*one is shown expanded in the insert at the left*). Each "spike" is only a few millivolts in height because this extracellular recording does not reflect the full transmembrane voltage change. Note that this neuron is firing at a nonzero "background rate" in the absence of stimuli, a trait typical of mammalian neurons. The stimulus that excites the neuron occurs for 0.5 second in this generic example. There is a burst of activity when the stimulus starts, decreasing to a rate above background for the stimulus duration.

In contrast to a microelectrode, a micropipette does not have a central, conducting wire. Instead, the fine-tipped pipette is filled with a conducting salt solution that allows it to record from inside a neuron that is carefully penetrated. Then, it can show all of the small voltage changes that occur, such as synaptic potentials, in addition to the action potential. Another type of micropipette with a specially polished tip is used to seal off and record from a tiny patch of neuronal membrane (thus, its name, *patch clamp*), allowing observation of the activity of individual membrane channels.

The strength and weakness of microelectrode and micropipette recording are the same: They allow us to study only one or a few neurons at a time. This specificity gives valuable information about the response properties of the neuronal building blocks of the nervous system. However, recording only a few cells at a time is a poor way to study how a system of multitudes of interacting neurons is accomplishing its task.

ELECTROENCEPHALOGRAPHY

An EEG allows the electrical activity of large groups of neurons to be studied simultaneously. It is

based on the fact that voltage changes in neurons give rise to extracellular current flow. When many neurons in a region are active, their combined extracellular current flow causes voltage changes that can be recorded with large electrodes placed on the surface of the skull.

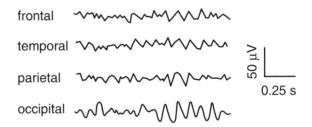

This figure shows simultaneous EEG records from four different electrode placements. No intentional stimuli are occurring; thus, background activity in a resting subject is being studied. In this situation there is significant synchrony in overall firing, giving rise to a somewhat regular pattern of voltage changes. The frequency of such rhythms varies in characteristic ways as a function of alertness.

When recording with only a few EEG electrodes, it is not possible to determine where in the brain the activity is occurring. However, note in the figure above that although the activity patterns in each recording are similar, there are differences in the voltages recorded at different skull positions, indicating regional variation. To take advantage of these variations, a large array of electrodes is used.

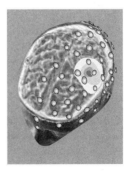

In this computer-generated result, the voltage recorded from multiple electrodes (*gray disks*) is shown as current density mapped onto the brain's surface. The stimulus was a touch on the skin, and the activity (*dark*

blue is highest) is appropriately mapped over the somatosensory region of the cortex.

MAGNETOENCEPHALOGRAPHY

An MEG monitors transient magnetic fields that result from neuronal activity. It is similar to an EEG because both record effects due to the overall current flows in the brain that result from neuronal activity. The MEG makes use of the fact that the time-varying currents cause tiny, localized magnetic fluctuations. The apparatus used to record the MEG (left) is at the cutting edge of modern technology, typically recording from an array of over 100 points across the entire skull. The device is usually inside a magnetically shielded room because artifacts easily override the small signal of about 0.25 microtesla (μT).

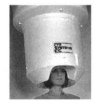 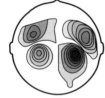 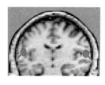

The computer-generated result of an experiment in which tones were played to both ears is shown here (*center*). Two magnetic dipoles are present, one on each side of the brain. (*Denser color indicates stronger fluctuations: blue, positive; black, negative.*) What is desired is to translate these data into a picture of the exact location in the brain where the activity arose. The determination involves a calculation that has more than one possible solution. Thus, information from EEG or fMRI studies is used to narrow the choices. The picture (*right*) shows the regions in the auditory cortex (*blue*) that were calculated as active when tones were sounded, superimposed on a MRI image.

SUMMARY AND COMPARISON

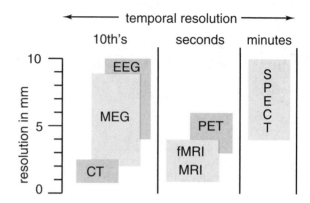

This figure compares the spatial and temporal characteristics of the various techniques. From a spatial point of view, it would seem that CT should always be used. However, it is important to remember that it does not differentiate soft tissue very well. EEG and MEG seem to give the best chance to visualize quickly occurring brain activity. However, they generally have a lower resolution than fMRI and PET, as well as problems of interpretation.

It is no surprise that fMRI and PET are now widely used, given their reasonable resolution both in time and in space. PET has the advantage of being able to visualize the localization of neurotransmitters and other neurochemicals of interest, but its expensive need for a nearby cyclotron limits its availability to a narrow group of researchers. This need is one reason why SPECT is more widely used, even though it cannot provide a good picture of the temporal order of events.

The figure does not show microelectrode, micropipette, and patch clamp recordings because they are off the scale, far to the left, and at the bottom due to their millisecond and micrometer resolution. These techniques are fundamentally different from those included in the figure, in that they allow and are limited to the study of only one or a few neurons at a time.

Perhaps the key point to take away is the complementary nature of all these techniques. Used together, they allow us to develop a conceptual picture of brain function.

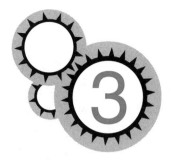

SENSING

REVIEW

Lecture 2 introduced the most common techniques used to visualize and study the functional anatomy of the brain. Tomographic reconstruction is a key concept in many of the visualization techniques. Tomography involves acquiring information about individual, adjacent thin sections of a structure and then using a computer to synthesize the information into a three-dimensional representation of the entire structure. Computed tomography (CT) scanning uses x-rays to build its pictures. However, the brain is soft tissue that poorly absorbs x-rays; thus, only very gross images can be obtained. These are most useful for locating dense tumors, foreign bodies, and fluid build-up in the brain due to internal bleeding.

Magnetic resonance imaging (MRI) provides excellent pictures of brain tissue by combining tomography with the atomic properties of the nuclei of individual atoms when exposed to magnetic fields. By manipulation of MRI parameters, both gray and white matter and the fluid-filled ventricles can be distinguished easily in great detail. This technique is extended in the process called functional MRI (fMRI), which can be used to study the activity of localized regions of the brain on a time scale of a few seconds. The brain of either a normal or impaired individual can be examined with fMRI while the subject is awake and performing some mental task. A related technique called positron emission tomography (PET) scanning is more limited because it uses short-lived radioactive compounds. However, it does allow particular molecules such as individual neurotransmitters to be localized. The use of these techniques in humans, starting in the 1990s, has revolutionized our understanding of how the human brain functions.

Electroencephalography (EEG) and magnetoencephalography (MEG) each combine tomography and the recording of currents in the brain resulting from the activity of groups of neurons. These techniques do not have the spatial resolution of MRI or PET, but can study events in real-time on a sub-millisecond time scale. Neurons can also be studied individually by recording from then using microelectrodes. This allows a fine-grained analysis of how individual neurons function. However, the technique is invasive and thus normally is used only in experiments that involve animals.

Sensory systems are the basis of knowing what is happening. This lecture begins with a presentation of some shared principles of their function. Then, individual sensory systems are explored, with special emphasis on the visual system because it is the best understood.

Next, similarities of visual and auditory parallel processing are highlighted. The most famous example of mapping, the somatosensory homunculus, is described. Finally, similarities in the taste and smell systems are discussed.

COMMON ORGANIZATIONAL PRINCIPLES

TRANSDUCTION

One neuron is much like another and action potentials are alike. So, how do we know the difference between green and salty? To answer this, we must understand how sensory receptors function. Everything that is sensed is a physical event that needs to be converted into the currency of the nervous system—

action potentials. This process, called *transduction*, is carried out by specialized nerve cells, the sensory receptors.

For example, photons of light are captured by rod and cone photoreceptors in the retina. Analogously, sound pressure is transduced by specialized hair cells in the ear. It is the specialization of these receptors that leads to separation of the senses; the hair cells in the cochlea do not react to photons of light, and retinal photoreceptors do not respond to sound pressure. Thus, the brain interprets action potentials from the eye as signals of light and those from the cochlea as signals of sound. One way to demonstrate this fact is to stimulate axons directly and determine what the subject experiences. If the human optic nerve is electrically stimulated, the subject "sees" light just as if the artificially initiated action potentials were the result of photoreceptor activity.

Put another way, we can say that the auditory and optic axons are *labeled lines*; one set is labeled for sounds, the other for sight. This separation is maintained as the signals are passed along a chain of neurons to sensory cortical regions and then to higher processing centers throughout the brain. Of course, different types of sensations are integrated at higher cortical levels but in ways that usually keep the sensation of salty from being green.

Interlude—*Synesthesia*

Synesthesia (from root words meaning "joined sensation") is a genetically determined condition experienced by about one in 25,000 people. For people with synesthesia, some sense experiences have multiple sensations. For example, hearing a word also elicits a sensation of color, or seeing blue also evokes a reproducible taste such as sweet. This unusual sensation does not require an act of will and is a consistent sensory experience. For a particular person usually only one sense type elicits an abnormal counterpart.

Synesthesia is idiosyncratic; a sound that is green to one synesthetic may be red to another. Their experiences seem perfectly normal to them, and they are surprised when they learn that most folks do not have such mixed sensations. Synesthetics often have exceptional memories that seem to be aided by their condition. For example, one reported recalling a

person because "she had a green name." Synesthetic experiences can be transiently elicited in about 5% of the normal population by electrical stimulation of the limbic system, a part of the brain usually associated with emotions.

Does synesthesia violate the principle of labeled lines? Neurologic examination suggests that synesthetics have significantly decreased activity in the more recently evolved regions of the left hemisphere and enhanced activity in the phylogenetically older limbic system, a brain area associated with emotion. It has been suggested that this imbalance, rather than an abnormal mixing of sensory pathways, is the basis of synesthesia. If so, it suggests that some degree of synesthesia occurs in all persons but only is unmasked and revealed to consciousness in synesthetics.

DECUSSATION

The left side of the body is dealt with by the right hemisphere of the brain and vice versa. For example, touch receptors in the skin on the right side of the body synapse with neurons that travel up the spinal cord and cross over to the left hemisphere of the brain. Such crossing is termed *decussation*.

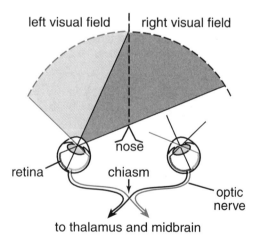

The situation is subtly different for vision, as depicted here. (*Visual field details are shown only for the left eye, for the sake of clarity.*) Each eye sees both the left and the right side of the world because our eyes are frontally placed. However, nerves from the left eye do not pass to the right hemisphere and those from the right eye do not pass to the left hemisphere. Rather, the retinal axons in the left eye's optic nerve that deal with the left side of the world cross over at a structure called the *optic chiasm* and terminate on the right side of the brain. Those that deal with the right side of the world do not cross, thus terminating on the left side. Axons in the right eye's optic nerve cross in a similar (but reversed) manner. Why there is decussation of sensory inputs is unknown. No theory of brain function demands it. It may simply be the result of an evolutionary accident.

THALAMIC RELAY

Sensory receptors project via a short chain of neurons to a specific location in the thalamus, each sense to its own location. (Smell is an exception; the projection is directly from the nose to the olfactory cortex.) Thalamic relay neurons carry the signal from there to the appropriate sensory cortical region. The thalamus is a gatekeeper in these pathways. It receives input back from the cortex that can cause one sense to be focused on while turning down the input from others. The thalamus also receives input from sleep centers that can turn down all sensory input to the cortex during sleep.

Terminology note: The thalamic region that receives input from one sense is called a *nucleus* (abbreviated "n"). This use of the word *nucleus* does not refer to the part of a cell that contains the DNA. Rather, it refers to a local group of neurons with a common function.

PARALLEL PROCESSING

A typical stimulus has multiple, characteristic factors. For example, a visual stimulus may have color, shape, intensity, spatial position, and movement. An auditory stimulus is usually characterized by parameters such as frequency, loudness, position, and duration. The multiple parameters of a stimulus are not analyzed altogether and in one place in the brain. Rather, one aspect is handled by one part of the appropriate sensory cortical region, another in another part, and so on. In addition, the different characteristics are

not analyzed sequentially, such as first shape, then color, and then position. Instead, the analysis of different aspects of the stimulus goes on simultaneously in adjacent sensory regions. The name given to this phenomenon is *parallel processing*. It is an important and general feature of all sensory systems.

VISION

RETINA

The retina does more than sense light. It is the initial visual-processing center of the brain. It consists of a thin, transparent layer of neurons and glial cells that lines the inside surface of the eyeball. Embryologically, it is actually brain tissue and its location makes it one of the easiest parts of the brain to study.

Retinal rod and cone photoreceptors (PR) have a region called the *outer segment* that contains specialized molecules, the *opsins*, that capture and transduce photons of light into changes in membrane voltage. Rods contain rhodopsin and are used for night vision. The brain translates their messages as black, white, or shades of gray. Humans and monkeys have three types of cones, each maximally responsive to different wavelengths: those sensitive to long (reddish), medium (greenish), and short (bluish) wavelengths. Together they are the basis of color vision.

The signal that light has been absorbed does not go directly from the photoreceptors to the thalamus. Instead, a small network of neurons in the retina starts to analyze the signal before it leaves the eye. The

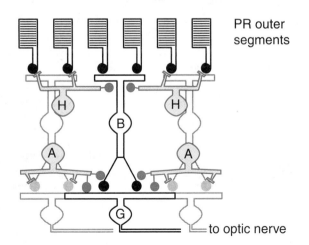

PR outer segments

to optic nerve

retina is depicted here in a very diagrammatic and highly simplified manner. (*Presynaptic terminals are shown as large, filled dots.*) The photoreceptors make synapses onto a neuron called a *bipolar cell* (B). Bipolar cells in turn synapse onto *ganglion cells* (G) whose axons leave the eye at the blind spot (optic disk) and form the optic nerve. Note that bipolar cells can collect input from more than one photoreceptor, and ganglion cells can have inputs from more than one bipolar cell. This retinal circuit, highlighted in black, thus can pool information. It also serves as the target for lateral interactions in the retina.

LATERAL INHIBITION

Lateral inhibition is a fundamental principle of brain organization. It is how neighboring neurons with related signals can influence each other and alter the nature of the information that is transmitted. The neurons that are the basis of this process in the retina are the horizontal (H) cells and the amacrine (A) cells (blue). Horizontal cells receive inputs from photoreceptors and carry this information laterally to bipolar cells. Amacrine cells carry information laterally from bipolar cells to other bipolar cells and to ganglion cells. The direct pathway through the retina (black) is influenced by what is going on in regions of the retina immediately surrounding it, via the lateral pathways. The lateral pathways are in blue to suggest that the lateral signal is of a different, inhibitory nature than the direct signal. Lateral interactions are a general feature of brain circuitry and are usually inhibitory.

Interlude—*Information*

How are parameters of a sensory stimulus, such as the brightness of a visual stimulus, encoded in the stream of action potentials that the stimulus causes? To answer this question, we need to understand one of the most important theoretical ideas in neuroscience, *information*. To start, think of a light switch that can be only *on* or *off*. It thus has two information states that convey all there is to know about its function. Another way to think of information is to consider bits in a digital computer. Each "0" or "1" that is part of the signal stream in a computer is a bit of information.

Everything that we know about the world is coded in streams of action potentials. Thus, action potentials both *signify* and *are* the basis of the brain's information. An individual action potential can be thought of as a single bit of information, so it is useful to use the language of physics, and to speak in terms of information when we discuss how neurons communicate with each other. For example, we say that information is *processed* as it moves through the brain, meaning that some aspect of the signal is emphasized as the action potentials in input neurons contribute to causing the firing of action potentials in their postsynaptic targets.

RECEPTIVE FIELDS

Every retinal ganglion cell is synaptically linked to a small, roughly circular patch of photoreceptors in the retina. That patch "looks" at a small region of space, owing to the optical nature of the eye. Changes in illumination in that spatial region can influence the ganglion cell's firing. The region is the "field of view" from which the ganglion cell receives input, and is called its *receptive field*. More generally for any neuron, its receptive field can be defined as the region in space where changes in the appropriate stimulus can significantly alter its firing rate.

What is meant by "space"? We readily know the answer for vision. It is not as obvious for the other senses. Auditory space is mainly the tonal quality of a stimulus. Touch space is a patch of skin. For taste and smell, space is defined by the "flavor" of molecules.

CENTER-SURROUND ORGANIZATION

A useful way to understand what any neuron "does" is to describe its receptive field in functional terms by determining the detailed nature of the stimuli that influence its firing. The next figure depicts two different ganglion cells as examples. The top part shows the spatial region where stimuli can influence each cell's response. Beneath each picture are graphs of the cell's firing rate for a period of about 2 seconds. The diagram between the graphs shows the stimulus that caused each response. For the top row the stimulus is a small spot of white light centered on the cell's receptive field. (*That is, the spot covers the dark blue, center region*

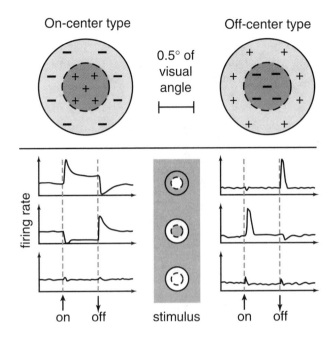

that the ganglion cell is most responsive to small but not large spots.

Terminology note: Visual receptive fields are measured in degrees of solid angle so that distance of a stimulus from the eye does not need to be stated. For example, the moon is about 0.5° wide, about the size of the center region of a typical receptive field.

COLOR CODING

The fovea is the small, central region of the retina used to discern fine detail. Foveal ganglion cells in humans and most primates receive inputs from only one or a few cones. The center-surround distinction for these ganglion cells not only is "On" versus "Off" but also is color-coded. Some ganglion cells are green-On-center/red-Off-surround while others are red-On-center/green-Off-surround. Other color pairs also exist. Thus, these ganglion cells not only are the basis of fine spatial discriminations because their center is fed by a small number of cones, but also are the basis for color vision.

Ganglion cells in the rest of the retina are predominantly rod-driven and have large non-color-coded receptive fields that are especially sensitive to moving and quickly changing stimuli. Here is a functional way to such receptive field organization: Most of our retina is specialized to notice that something new is happening in regions that are away from the center of gaze. The resulting ganglion cell activity signals certain brain centers to move our eyes and focus our foveas on the target to examine that "something" in detail.

PARALLEL PROCESSING IN THE VISUAL SYSTEM

About one-third of the brain is used to process the visual signal, more than for any other sensory function. The processing occurs in a highly organized and interconnected manner, as depicted in the next diagram. The diagram is purposely complex to convey the complexity of what is happening when we see. Yet, it shows only a few of the more than 25 cortical areas that deal with vision.

Two main pathways are emphasized in bold print. The primary pathway that is involved in analysis

shown in the receptive field pictures.) In the middle row the stimulus is an annulus of white light that covers only the surround (*light blue region*) of each receptive field. The bottom stimulus is a large, white spot that falls simultaneously on the center and the surround.

The ganglion cell on the left is a sustained responding "On-center" type because its firing rate increases above the background rate when the centered spot of light goes on (up arrow). This increase is signified by plus (+) signs in the receptive field picture. The ganglion cell on the right is a transiently responding "Off-center" type. Its firing rate increases when the centered spot of light goes off (down arrow), signified by the minus (−) signs in its receptive field center. Note that its firing rate actually decreases during the presence of the light. (An analogous decrease occurs when light goes off for the On-center cell.) The response of each cell reverses when an annulus of light covers only its surround. The On-center cell has an "Off" surround, and the Off-center one has an "On" surround.

What happens when the center and surround are stimulated simultaneously, as shown in the bottom row? There is very little response when the light goes on or off because the excitatory and inhibitory phases of the responses from each region cancel each other out. Such cancellation is an example of lateral inhibition, where the region that surrounds the receptive field center—the region lateral to it—has a response antagonistic to the center's response. What purpose does lateral inhibition serve in this case? One function is to ensure

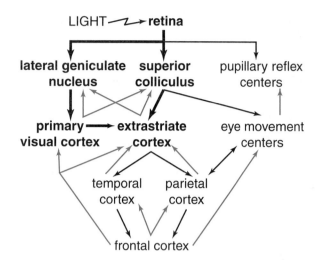

feedback to the extrastriate cortex that relates specifically to the facial features of that image. The feedback causes extrastriate cortical cells to filter out other details and concentrate on just the face.

RECEPTIVE FIELD COMPLEXITY

Receptive fields in the cortex have properties that are more complex than those in primary sensory areas such as the retina. Typically, a small number of spatially adjacent LGN inputs synapse with each neuron in V1. There they are recombined to emphasize features of the visual image.

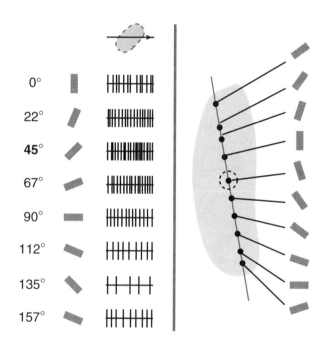

of the visual scene goes from the retina to the lateral geniculate nucleus (LGN) to the primary visual cortex (called *striate cortex* because of its appearance in anatomic sections, and also called *V1* and *area 17*). The LGN is a thalamic relay nucleus and is a predominant gateway to the cortex, as are most thalamic nuclei. A small amount of processing occurs in the LGN; however, the major analysis of the image starts in the V1, where the LGN inputs are combined. From there, the signal passes to higher processing centers in the occipital lobe and then to regions specialized for visual processing in the parietal and temporal lobes. The second major stream of information flow through the visual system is from the retina to the superior colliculus, a region of the tectum. The signal is then relayed to cortical regions that have to do with moving the eyes to focus on a specific point in space.

A general principal exemplified by these multiple pathways is that the job of image analysis is divided into parallel streams with differing functions. These subdivisions of the visual pathway deal with their tasks simultaneously, allowing analysis to be done more quickly than if it was carried out sequentially.

Another principle illustrated in the visual pathway diagram is *feedback*, also called *top-down influence*. The blue arrows in the above figure indicate that cortical centers send signals back to the same regions that provide their input. Such feedback allows what is being communicated at a given moment to be influenced by processing of what has been signaled immediately before it. For example, a region in the temporal lobe decodes images of the human face. It also sends

One example of the many types of specialized receptive fields is illustrated on the left side of this figure. It shows a neuron that responds best to a moving dark bar. The oval-shaped receptive field (*blue*) is pictured at the top. The arrow depicts the direction and path taken by the bar. Eight different passes through the field are shown, with the bar at a different angle during each pass. The response of the neuron as the bar passes through the receptive field is also shown. This particular cell responds best when the bar is oriented at 45°. It responds less vigorously the further from 45° the bar is tilted, and only at the background rate when the bar is oriented at 135° (perpendicular to the optimum orientation). A subset of these neurons is also direction-ally sensitive; if the best oriented bar is moved in the direction opposite to that shown by the arrow, a cell this is directionally sensitive does not respond.

The right side of the figure illustrates that such orientation-sensitive neurons are not arrayed randomly in the cortex. A patch of visual cortex (*blue*) a few millimeters long is shown viewed from above. Neurons in this part of the cortex were sampled along the blue line at the black points, and their best orientation was determined as pictured on the far right. Note that neurons in adjacent regions have receptive fields with best orientations that differ by only a few degrees. Also, all orientations are present in a gradually changing, regular array.

The dashed circle calls attention to another important point. It indicates the top of a column of cells that lies perpendicular to the surface, passing through the entire thickness of the cortical gray matter. All of the cells in such a *cortical column* have receptive fields with the same preferred orientation, although other of their properties can be different. These two principles are typical of sensory cortical regions: (1) laterally adjacent areas respond to related but systematically differing best stimuli; (2) all of the cells in a local column have closely related receptive fields. Having adjacent cells deal with related parts of the image facilitates synaptic and functional interactions.

WHAT AND WHERE

The features, color, and position of a stimulus are dealt with in parallel in different cortical regions. This figure of the brain's left hemisphere viewed from the rear shows the physical relationships of some of

these areas. Primary visual cortex (V1) is bordered on the medial face by area V2 (*dark gray*), the first of the extrastriate visual areas in the occipital lobe. Each of the areas V1 through V5 has its own complete retinotopic map. (*V3, V4, and V5 are not specifically labeled.*) The presence of repeated maps is one of the ways that these areas can be defined as distinct from each other. Their sequential names reflect the fact that they are somewhat hierarchical, with each providing streams of input to the next. Yet, especially past V3, they also are involved in parallel processing of the visual signal, with different aspects of the stimulus being emphasized. For example, most of the neurons in V5 deal with the color information in the visual image.

The outputs of occipital regions V1 through V5 provide multiple streams of input to many cortical areas in the temporal and parietal lobes that deal with vision. These pathways exemplify the full splendor of parallel processing. The parietal areas deal mainly with *where* images are in space. Thus, the participating areas are termed the "where" stream of the visual pathways. The temporal cortical regions are organized to analyze the form of the objects that make up the visual image, comprising the "what" stream. An especially interesting area in the right temporal lobe of humans and some other primates contains neurons that respond specifically to faces and facial features. Its existence probably reflects the fact that faces are critical to the social recognition that is at the heart of primate societies.

If different parts of the cortex deal with the analysis of different aspects of the visual image, where is it all put back together? Is there a virtual "movie screen" somewhere in the brain where all of this careful analysis is recombined into a nice picture? Besides raising the question of "who" is watching the movie screen, this question reflects an old, mechanistic view of how the brain might be organized. Now we know that there is no final viewing screen. Rather, the moment-to-moment, simultaneous activity of the neurons throughout the visual areas of the brain is the only basis for knowing what we are seeing.

The concept of simultaneous processing of different aspects of the visual scene in different cortical regions leads to the question of how the color information in one place, the form information in another, and the motion analysis in still another region are accurately associated. Why are not the colors of a flag sometimes "put" onto the wrong stripes? This issue is called the *binding problem* because it addresses the question of

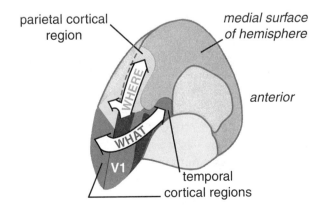

parietal cortical region

medial surface of hemisphere

WHERE

anterior

WHAT

V1

temporal cortical regions

how the common properties of parts of an image stay perceptually bound together although they are analyzed separately. It is currently the subject of much study and speculation.

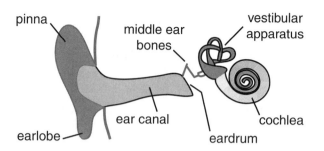

Interlude—*Prosopagnosia*

Bill Choisser writes, "I met my mother on the sidewalk and did not recognize her. We walked towards each other, and passed within two feet. . . . The only way I know about this is because she told me about it that night. She was not amused at all by this incident, and she has never forgiven me for it." Bill is one of a small number of people born without the ability to recognize faces. This is called *prosopagnosia*, although he uses the term *face blindness*.

Face-blind individuals can see faces; they just cannot recognize them. Some people acquire the condition after a stroke or injury that damages the region in the right temporal lobe responsible for face recognition. Severity varies, although the dysfunction can be so severe that when looking at two photographs of the same face, the individual simply does not recognize they are the same. It is not that prosopagnosics simply cannot tell one person from another; they are able to identify people based on their voice or nonfacial features. Because we now understand that recognition of faces is localized to its own special region of the temporal visual stream, it is not surprising that injuries or developmental deficits involving that region can lead to this remarkably specific perceptual difficulty.

HEARING

EAR

Humans can hear accurately over an extremely wide range of intensities, from the movement of a few air molecules in a sound-deadened room to the roar of a nearby jet engine. Our range of frequency discrimination is similarly broad, from 20 Hz, a bass deep enough to feel, to 20,000 Hz, a pitch so high we may wonder if we are really hearing something (*Hz=Hertz=cycles/sec*). The design of the ear is basic to accomplishing these feats. The outer ear consists of what may seem like two

pieces of irrelevant anatomy, the thing stuck to the side of your head (called the *pinna*), and the place where wax collects, the *ear canal*. Both, however, are superb acoustic devices, specifically shaped to capture and channel the broad range of sound we can hear.

The ear canal ends at the eardrum, which vibrates the three delicate bones of the middle ear. These then vibrate the oval window of the fluid-filled cochlea. A direct interface between vibrating air and the water-filled cochlea would be a very poor one for transferring changing pressures. Instead, the movements of the bones of the middle ear accomplish that job. They also have attached muscles that can decrease the transmission of potentially damaging loud sounds, acting in response to feedback from the brain.

COCHLEA

The vestibular apparatus, which is used to sense balance and motion, and the cochlea comprise the inner ear. The cochlea is spiral-shaped and has a complex inner structure that is the neurosensory apparatus for hearing. Sensory neurons named *hair cells* are the transduction site. Their "hairs" are actually specialized cilia attached to membranes within the cochlea that vibrate in response to sound vibrations. The mechanical deformation of the hair cell membranes leads to conductance changes and to synaptic transmission to the neurons, whose axons then become the eighth cranial nerve.

The cochlea is organized tonotopically. High frequencies cause vibrations at its basal end (*light blue in the ear figure*); low frequencies cause vibrations of its apical end (*dark blue*), with intermediate frequencies falling smoothly in between. Thus, each hair cell becomes a frequency-labeled line. Its receptive field is the narrow range of sound frequencies that each one is sensitive to. The cochlea receives feedback from brain neurons that can attenuate its frequency sensitivity.

This feedback sharpens attention to momentarily relevant sounds at the expense of others.

PARALLEL PROCESSING IN THE AUDITORY SYSTEM

Just as the visual system must deal with multiple features such as shape, color, position, and movement, the auditory system must simultaneously decode numerous aspects of sound including loudness, pitch, and harmonics, as well as the timing of multiple sounds and where they are coming from. Again, parallel processing is the rule, although in this sensory system much of it occurs below the level of the cortex. Only the basics are shown in the next figure. The full complexity includes inputs from both ears as well as feedback circuits.

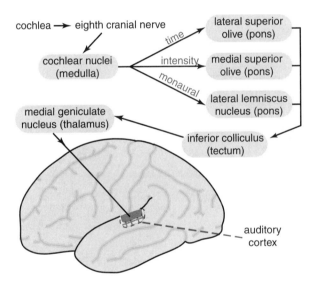

A sound that does not originate from the exact midline reaches the ears at slightly different times. Although the time difference is only tens of microseconds, neurons in the lateral superior olivary (LSO) nucleus are tuned to respond to it. Thus, the firing of each LSO neuron corresponds to a different point in space where sound can originate. Above 3 kHz, the auditory system makes use of the fact that for higher frequencies the head is an effective sound blocker. Thus, a sound off to one side provides a louder signal to one ear than to the other. Neurons in the medial superior olivary nucleus are tuned to respond to these

intensity differences. The pathway through the lateral lemniscus is monaural and seems to deal with determining when sounds start and stop and with other properties that do not depend on a sound's position in space.

All of these streams of information project to and interact in the inferior colliculus where further analysis takes place. Then the signal is relayed through the gatekeeper thalamus to the auditory cortex. The first two areas of that cortex, A1 and A2, are in the superior temporal gyrus of the temporal lobe. Part of the auditory cortex (*dark blue*) lies on the lateral surface, but much (*light-gray crosshatch*) is buried within the sylvian sulcus. Major output from the auditory cortical areas is to nearby regions that deal with language, which is discussed in Lecture 5.

An important point about the auditory system relates to auditory receptive fields. All neurons in the system respond to some sound frequencies (tones) better than others. However, as information moves through the auditory system, neurons are increasingly narrowly tuned to specific frequencies and intensities.

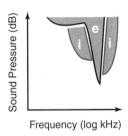

The figure shows a representative receptive field for such a neuron, called a *tuning curve*. The gray areas show frequencies and intensities that the neuron responds to in an excitatory (*e*) manner, in this case most sharply and sensitively to a relatively high frequency. Flanking bands that provide inhibitory (*i*) inputs (*blue*) in a type of lateral inhibition help tune the response to a narrow frequency range.

TOUCH AND PAIN

SENSORY RECEPTORS

All touch does not elicit the same sensation. We can differentiate objects based on texture, vibration, shape, and pressure. Pain can be sharp, deep, burning, or itching. The initial basis of such diversity is found in the structure of touch and pain sensory receptors. Sensory receptors for different aspects of touch and pain have different responses based on their structure.

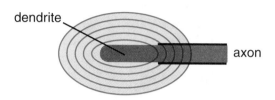

Touch receptors respond to physical deformation of their specialized dendritic-like ending and are called *mechanoreceptors*. The figure shows one type, the Pacinian corpuscle. Its core is a single dendrite that changes conductance when stretched and then initiates an action potential at its base. Surrounding the dendrite is an onion-like, nonneuronal structure of fluid-filled sacs. When initially deformed by a mechanical stimulus, the sacs physically transfer the deformation to the dendrite, initiating an action potential. Removal of the stimulus also causes a momentary deformation and action potential. However, during the continuous portion of any stimulus the fluid between the layers redistributes and physically damps out the mechanical pressure on the dendrite. Thus, the Pacinian corpuscle only signals changes in touch—start and stop—not continuous pressure.

Other mechanoreceptors have different structural specializations that lead to their specificity as labeled lines for different types of touch. Pain receptors (synonym: *nociceptors*) have bare, dendritic-like endings that respond to excessive, potentially damaging mechanical deformation or to noxious chemicals. Thermoreceptors change conductance and firing rate in response to heating and cooling.

SENSORY HOMUNCULUS

Touch, pain, and temperature information reaches the cortex via complex, parallel pathways through the spinal cord to midbrain nuclei and the thalamus. The picture shows the primary (S1, *light blue*) and secondary (S2, *dark blue*) somatic sensory areas in the cortex. Most of S2 is not visible because it is buried

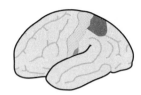

in the sulcus. S3, just anterior to S1, is also buried. Adjacent to S1 is a region of parietal lobe (*gray*) that receives outputs from S1 and S2.

S1 itself is subdivided into multiple regions, each with its own map. These maps represent another case of parallel processing. The regions receive separate projections of different aspects of somatic sensation such as rapidly adapting stimuli, deep stimuli, fine discrimination, and pain location. S1 and S2 have outputs that project to subcortical areas to provide feedback that causes selective attention to some stimuli at the expense of others.

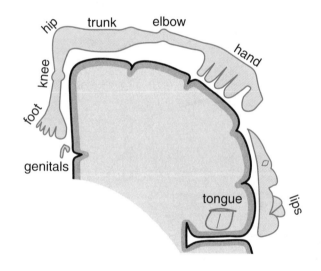

The S1 cortical somatotopic map provides the most vivid example of the mapping concept. The figure shows a coronal section through S1 (in the right hemisphere) and indicates the parts of the body surface that are represented at various parts of the cortical surface. For example, the top medial edge of S1 corresponds to the hip region. Such diagrams were originally made from studies of sensory deficits in people after strokes and by using microelectrode recording in monkeys. Recently, the details have been extended using MEG.

The amount of cortex devoted to a particular body region is represented schematically by the size of that region in the diagram of the body (*blue*). The entire picture is called a *homunculus*. Its most interesting feature is that it is not uniform, reflecting the fact that some parts of the body have much finer touch discrimination and sensation than others. Not surprisingly, there is a large amount of somatosensory cortex devoted to the fingers, our primary touch site for detecting shape and form. This specialization can be thought of as analogous to the large amount of visual cortex devoted to the most important retinal region, the fovea, that is involved in making fine visual discriminations. Other areas that have remarkably expanded representation are the toes and lips. It is easy to imagine evolutionary explanations for these specializations.

Interlude—*It Hurts Where?*

A patient reported to the doctor that she had a dull, intermittent pain between her shoulder blades. She took aspirin and applied rubbing ointments for muscle injury, but they did not help. Taking time off from her exercise program was of no use. The pain returned when she started again.

Pain is a complex phenomenon dealt with by multiple parallel systems. Sharp pain, such as from stepping on a tack, is usually brief, intense, and easily localized. It is transmitted up the spinal cord to the brain via a pathway of fast-conducting axons. Deep, dull pain, such as from a stomachache, is usually hard to localize and can be long-lasting. It is transmitted via a different pathway of slow-conducting axons. Those axons often have numerous sensory endings that terminate in a very wide region within the viscera of the body. This pattern of innervation can make it easier to know that something hurts rather than *where* exactly the pain comes from.

Given these facts, her physician suspected that the pain in her back was "referred pain" and correctly diagnosed gallstones. Referred pain occurs because the activity of the visceral, slow-conducting fibers activates touch receptors on the skin in a nearby region as well as the deep-pain pathway. Thus, the pain was being caused by her gallbladder (next to the liver), but felt like it was coming from near her shoulder blades, a common symptom. Strain due to exercise was not her problem; rather, digestion of the meals she ate after exercising was causing pain from temporary enlargement of gallstones.

TASTE AND SMELL

Taste and smell are termed "chemical senses" because the binding of individual molecules excites their sensory receptors. It is appropriate to discuss them together not only for this reason, but also because they interact at cortical levels. The interaction is best exemplified by the notion of "flavor." When a tasty food is eaten, the flavor sensation requires activation of taste buds on the tongue and nasal odor receptors. This is easily demonstrated by blocking each in turn and observing how the richness of a complex flavor is diminished.

The tasks of these senses are varied, including social recognition via odor and pheromones, food selection, and avoidance of toxins. Odors strongly evoke emotions, as discussed in Lecture 6. Most of these functions are more highly developed in animals below the primate level that do not place as much reliance on vision as we do. Unfortunately, the systems' long evolutionary pedigree is not matched by our understanding of how they function. The basic problem is that the stimuli are hard to characterize; the "shape" of a molecule is less readily defined than the wavelength of light or sound.

RECEPTORS

Is there a taste bud with a unique receptor for each different taste we can discern? Is there an olfactory receptor for each distinct odor? Probably not. We can discriminate about 2000 different odors and perhaps 1000 different tastes. This ability is partly accomplished by a large number of unique receptor sites built into taste buds and olfactory receptors. However, research shows that an individual receptor in either of these systems responds to more than one molecular type.

In the tongue, the sensations of sweet, sour, salty, and bitter tend to be predominant in any one taste bud but are not totally segregated. Further, there is evidence for a small number of different receptors sensitive to each of these four taste categories. Strong evidence exists for a fifth taste category, *umami* ("delicious taste"). This is the taste of monosodium-l-glutamate (MSG), which is extensively used in the cooking of some Asian cultures. Neurons have been found in gustatory areas of the cortex that are selectively responsive to MSG applied to the tongue, and a glutamate receptor in certain taste buds is suggested to be the basis of this fifth taste category. However, some researchers challenge even the concept of basic taste categories, judging that the overlap of sensitivities of individual gustatory neurons is too extensive for simple characterization.

Recently, a few genetic mutations associated with taste deficiencies in humans have been mapped. The localization of such genes suggests that the ultimate unraveling of the human genome may be the only way to settle the controversy that surrounds the concept of basic taste categories.

Odors are even harder to characterize into groups than are tastes, so much so that researchers do not agree on a single set of "primary odors." In fact, studies show that different cultures describe different sets of primary odors. This classification problem is consistent with the large number of different odor receptors that have been identified.

Given the mixing of sensitivities at the basic transduction level, how is our ability to discern odors and tastes accomplished? A visual analogy serves as a good starting point in answering this question. Our retina has only three different types of cones, each with broadly overlapping wavelength sensitivities. Yet, we can distinguish thousands of different colors. Each "color" activates a unique amount of activity in each cone type. Analysis of these combinations at cortical levels underlies our color perceptions. Similarly, complex analysis of the combined output of many different specific receptors is probably the basis for discrimination in our chemical senses.

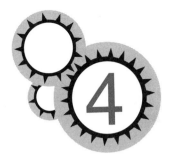

ACTING

REVIEW

The previous lecture presented the way information from the world gets to our brain via the senses. Initially a sensory receptor such as a photoreceptor, a touch sensor, a cochlear hair cell, or a chemoreceptor transduces the physical stimulus into a voltage change in a neuron. Then, action potentials carry a message of the stimulus throughout the brain. The brain interprets stimuli as the "correct" sense according to where the input occurs: eye=light, ear=sound, etc.

The signals from all senses except smell pass through a relay center in the thalamus before reaching the cortex. The thalamus acts as gatekeeper, allowing concentration on one sense at a time. Once sensory information reaches the cortex it is split into multiple parallel streams that are dealt with simultaneously by multiple brain regions. This method of dealing with inputs is called parallel processing.

The retina does more than simply relay signals about light and dark. In fact, the retina is a small piece of the brain with numerous cell types organized into networks that begin the analysis of the visual signal. Cells in two of the retinal layers communicate in a lateral direction across the retina, usually inhibiting and sharpening other retinal activity.

The retinal networks result in concentric, center-surround–type receptive fields at the ganglion cell level. Ganglion cell axons then transmit this processed information to the rest of the brain via the optic nerve. In the cortex the visual signal is analyzed in parallel streams of cortical sites that deal either with the "what" or "where" of the elements of the visual scene, an instance of parallel processing. Visual receptive fields of cortical neurons are more stimulus-specific than retinal ganglion cell receptive fields, and are organized in complex arrays, such as orientation columns, that mirror their function.

Parallel processing in the auditory system takes the tonotopic output of the cochlea of each ear and analyzes pitch, loudness, and spatial origin simultaneously. The receptive fields of neurons in the primary auditory cortex are most sensitive to certain pitches, not to spatial aspects of the signal.

The somatosensory system provides the most striking example of how aspects of the world are mapped onto the cortex. The homunculus is essentially an image of the body stretched over the somatic input areas. It is "distorted," with important areas such as the fingers occupying a relatively larger proportion of cortex than their small surface area relative to the rest of the body would predict.

Taste and smell are chemical senses based on the stereochemical interaction of molecules breathed in or taken into the mouth, with receptors in the nasal passages or on the tongue. There are only a few types of taste receptors and perhaps a few thousand different odor receptors. Gustatory experience is usually a combination of both the taste and odor of a particular food. The odor system is very primitive, in evolutionary terms, and the signals from the receptors do not pass through the thalamus. They go, instead, directly to the olfactory cortex and surrounding regions that deal with emotions.

All behaviors involve the action of muscles. All of the brain's output to the world is nothing but muscle contraction and relaxation. Be it an uncoordinated stumble, exquisite piano playing, scanning the horizon, or the uttering of words, the action of muscles is necessary and responsible. All of our thoughts and intentions—voluntary and involuntary—that become actions are transmitted to the world by movements of our muscles. So, it is not surprising that a significant amount of the brain is devoted to motor output tasks.

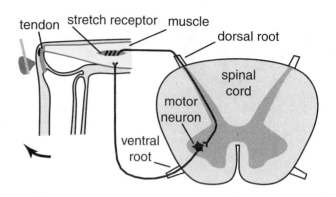

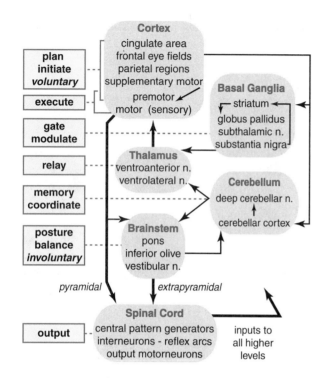

This figure summarizes the major components of the motor system. The actual interconnecting pathways are so profuse that a diagram showing them all would be confusingly covered with lines. The main point here is that the system consists of a hierarchy of interacting levels. The next sections discuss their main functions and relationships.

SPINAL CORD

Basic movement patterns reside in the spinal cord, as shown in the following example. The signal for a muscle to contract is a burst of action potentials that travel down the axons of *alpha motor neurons* to muscle fibers. The simplest activation of such a neuron is via a *reflex arc*. Muscles have specialized internal structures called *stretch receptors* that are buried deep inside them. In the example in this figure, a sensory stretch receptor in the quadriceps muscle of the leg sends its associated

axon to the spinal cord (*shown in cross section*) where it synapses onto the motor neuron. When the reflex-test hammer hits the patellar tendon, the tendon moves, pulling on the muscle. The stretch receptor within the muscle is elongated and sends a signal to the cord. This signal, in turn, causes the muscle to contract (shorten) in an attempt to counteract the unexpected stretch. Such a two-neuron reflex arc can be thought of as the most basic, built-in motor circuit that accomplishes a specific task.

Reflex pathways in the spinal cord can be more complex than the simple reflex arc, helping to coordinate the multiple muscles involved in a task. When a weight tries to push your hand down and your intent is to keep the forearm level, both of the muscles shown in this figure must work together.

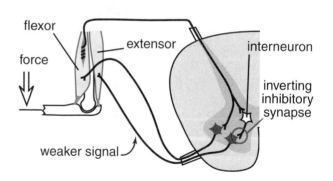

In response to signals from the stretch receptor, the flexor (agonist) in front must shorten while tension in the rear extensor (antagonist) must be decreased by removal of some excitation. Relaxation of the extensor is accomplished by interneurons that invert the muscle-spindle signal from excitatory to inhibitory, thus lessening the firing of the motor neuron that activates the extensor. Spinal cord circuits of greater complexity are used to coordinate the movement of many muscles, such as when you are walking. These circuits are called *central pattern generators*.

In all of these examples, the spinal cord neurons are considered in isolation to emphasize the important concept that many movements can have their basic form organized in the spinal cord. Of course, all of these circuits can be modulated by signals from the brain, as we will see next.

BRAINSTEM

Signals reach motor neurons via two pathways. One is directly from the cortex, mainly from neurons called pyramidal cells, and is named the *pyramidal tract*. It is mainly responsible for fine, voluntary movements. The other is a set of tracts from the brainstem that make up the *extrapyramidal tracts*. These are mainly responsible for overall posture and balance, usually controlled involuntarily such that you are unaware of how the exact muscle movements are carried out. The fact that these circuits are automatic is fortunate. You would not want to have to think about taking every breath. Moreover, you could not really consciously coordinate all the muscular and postural adjustments that occur moment by moment when you walk.

Interlude—*Ondine's Curse*

In an ancient French myth, a human lover spurned a mermaid. In retribution the god of the sea cursed him to have to think about every breath he took. Obviously, he then could do little else or he would die. Even sleep was virtually impossible. Unfortunately, a few babies are born yearly with this condition—called *Ondine's curse*—due to improper development of their neural breathing control centers. (*Ondine* is the French word for "mermaid.")

If the problem is quickly realized, the baby is put on a respirator, which is necessary forever. Recently, this horrible necessity has been removed by the development of a small implantable device that regularly shocks and thus excites the nerve trunk that causes contraction of the diaphragm, resulting in reasonably normal breathing.

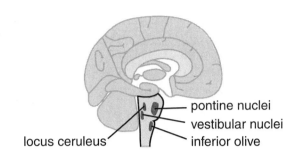

pontine nuclei
vestibular nuclei
inferior olive
locus ceruleus

Many brainstem nuclei are major sites that organize involuntary motor control. They are a main source of the input to and output from the cerebellum. The inferior olivary nucleus is a primary source of input to all cerebellar regions. The vestibular nuclei receive significant input from the vestibular apparatus in the inner ear and from the cerebellum. They have outputs to the spinal cord, which together with outputs from regions of the midbrain tegmentum and the pons ensures whole-body balance and posture. This control is basically reflexive and does not need conscious intervention. So, these sensory input–brainstem–spinal cord output pathways are referred to as *closed-loop circuits*.

BASAL GANGLIA

The basal ganglia, at the base of the cerebral cortex, play a pivotal gating role in allowing or inhibiting voluntary movements that are initiated by motor cortical regions. The diagram shows the basal ganglia

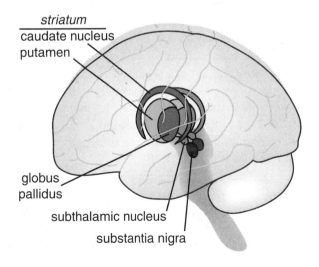

striatum
caudate nucleus
putamen
globus
pallidus
subthalamic nucleus
substantia nigra

and associated nuclei that are responsible for motor activities. Almost all inputs to the basal ganglia are from the cortex to the striatal nuclei, while most outputs are from portions of the globus pallidus and subthalamic nuclei. These mainly project back to the cortex via the ventroanterior (VA) and ventrolateral (VL) thalamic nuclei.

Terminology note: Technically speaking, the nuclei in gray and black in the figure are not part of the anatomically defined basal ganglia. Also, a major component of the basal ganglia, the amygdala, is not shown but will be discussed in Lecture 6, on emotions. Many authors refer to all of these structures as the basal ganglia, based on their functional association.

It is important to recognize that the basal ganglia do not organize movements or cause them via spinal cord projections, but rather are more like an important traffic cop in the voluntary movement paths. Two diseases highlight this gating function.

PARKINSON'S DISEASE AND HUNTINGTON'S DISEASE

The substantia nigra are a pair of nuclei that are a major source of dopamine-releasing neurons whose axons project to many cortical regions. A main target of these axons is the striatum. In Parkinson's disease the cells of the substantia nigra progressively degenerate, usually starting during middle age. Symptoms are related to motor activity: resting tremor that abates when voluntary movement is initiated; rigidity caused by simultaneous activation of agonist and antagonist muscles; posture, balance, and locomotion problems; and hypokinesia and bradykinesia. The latter provide an interesting insight into basal ganglia function. Hypokinesia is the inability to start an intended movement and the patient seems frozen in position. Once a movement does start, it seems to be carried out in slow motion (bradykinesia).

Early-stage Parkinson's is treated by having the patient take l-dopa, a metabolic precursor of dopamine. l-dopa helps increase the dopamine content of substantia nigra cells and thus boosts whatever dopamine release is still present. Eventually, this treatment loses effectiveness and other measures must

be taken. In later stages, surgery that destroys the brain regions responsible for excessive tremor is used as a palliative treatment. Recently, an exciting new therapy was developed. It involves the use of immature brain cells that are precursors of dopamine neurons. These are surgically implanted into the patient's basal ganglia where—remarkably—they actually make new dopamine-releasing synapses onto appropriate neurons and reduce symptoms.

Huntington's disease, caused by an autosomal dominant mutation, is due in part to degeneration of the caudate nucleus. Symptoms usually appear in middle age and are progressive, leading to death about 10 to 20 years later. The motor component of the disease involves involuntary, rapid, jerky movements (called *chorea*) of extremities, whole limbs, and facial and vocal musculature. Cognitive functions are eventually impaired as well. Although the gene mutation that causes the disease is known, no treatment yet exists.

Parkinson's disease shows how disruption of the normal gating functions of the basal ganglia interferes with starting and stopping movements. Similarly, Huntington's disease reveals inappropriate movements when the normal balance of controls in the basal ganglia fails.

OTHER DISEASES RELATED TO THE BASAL GANGLIA

It is predictable that diseases of the basal ganglia involve movement, but it is surprising that defects in learning, mental state, and cognitive diseases can also be traced to basal ganglia malfunction. These conditions show how intimately the motor aspects of behavior contribute to our overall mental state.

Obsessive-compulsive disorder (OCD) involves repeated, ritualistic behavior patterns that uselessly consume great amounts of time. The involvement of the basal ganglia in starting, stopping, and modulating the intensity of motor patterns provides a hint at how this region may be involved in OCD. Neuroimaging studies show hyperactivity in the caudate nucleus and putamen during OCD episodes, as well as in brain regions that interact with these areas such as the orbital cortex and cingulate gyrus. Such activity could reflect overactivation of behaviors otherwise maintained in proper balance by controls in the basal ganglia.

Various experiments show that the basal ganglia are involved in the shifting of attention from one activity or motor pattern to another. This fact helps us to understand the involvement of dopamine pathways in the basal ganglia in attention deficit and hyperactivity disorder (ADHD). Individuals with this condition have difficulty maintaining attention on a single task but instead constantly and inappropriately shift their attention around.

CORTEX AND THALAMUS

Lecture 3 discussed the fact that most sensory information reaches the cerebral cortex by way of relay centers in the thalamus. For the information that reaches the somatosensory cortex and generates the sensory homunculus, the relay is via the ventroposterior nucleus. The brainstem and cerebellum also project back to the cortex via the thalamic VA and VL nuclei. The interposition of the thalamus as a kind of gatekeeper in all of these pathways is important for allowing you to focus attention on one sensory system at a time, as well as for turning down all but the "loudest" inputs to the cortex during sleep.

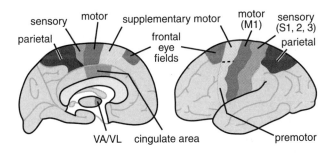

The portion of the cortex that is primarily responsible for the pyramidal pathway projections, the motor cortex (M1), lies immediately anterior to the central sulcus, parallel to the motor input in the somatic sensory (synonym: *somatosensory*) cortex (S1, 2, 3). It is organized into an output homunculus that basically mirrors the input homunculus discussed in Lecture 3, thus facilitating interconnections between the two. However, these two cortical regions do not strictly obey the principle that cortical sensory input and output regions are separate. Outputs to the spinal cord and some inputs can be found in both regions, as well as in the premotor cortex, which primarily feeds M1. This mixing makes the broader point that when systems are considered as a whole, the border between input and output is not sharp in any of the sensory modes.

THE SELF IN SPACE

Cortical regions adjacent to M1 and the somatosensory cortex are responsible for processing information relevant to movement that arises in any and all of the body systems. For example, a region of the parietal cortex (*shaded in the figure*) relays visual information that is important for knowing where the body and its parts are in space. That information, combined with processing in the frontal eye fields, is critical in coordinating eye movements, an obvious function for visual information. Perhaps less obvious is its role in supplying the knowledge of where things are when they are not in the direct field of view.

For example, you see a glass on an adjacent table and then look away. Then, without looking back at it, you reach for the glass and accurately pick it up. What part of the brain remembers where the glass is? Further, is the movement based on a body-centered system of coordinates or on an externally centered system of spatial coordinates? Studies of individual neurons in the premotor cortex of monkeys provide evidence to help answer these questions. Experiments revealed neurons that fired when an object was first touched. They then continued to fire when the target was no longer visible. Analysis showed that they encoded the target's position in a coordinate system that was centered on the head. Such neurons are part of an overall system that builds a stable, remembered map of the space that immediately surrounds the body. Other studies show that for objects that are out of your immediate reach, the coordinates of space that you use to localize them are centered on them, not you.

Even subtle details are stored in spatial memory. If you know that a big round object and a small thin one are within reach, when you reach for one of them in the dark, your hand automatically assumes the grasp appropriate for picking up the shape you are reaching for. All in all, "knowing where you are" is first a motor task that relates you to the immediate surroundings you must move in, and that involves the interaction of almost all your sensorimotor regions.

Interlude—*Spatial Hemineglect*

To move, you must know where you are and where in the immediate space around you that you are going. The right parietal cortex is critically important for this sense of self in space. A stroke involving the supramarginal gyrus of the right inferior parietal lobule can vividly reveal this function. (Recall that the right hemisphere deals with the left side of the world.) Such a stroke often results in *spatial hemineglect* in which patients deny the existence of the left half of objects, including the left side of their body, even though tests show their visual cortex still "sees" all of space. When looking at a whole scene, they ignore things on the left.

In one famous example, an artist with such a stroke drew a detailed picture of his town's main plaza as seen while facing west. Only buildings on his right side (north) were in the picture. When he then drew the same scene while facing east, again only buildings on his right side were included, but now these were the entirely different set of buildings to the south! Perhaps even more surprising, such patients deny they have any problem or that anything is wrong with their perception—an apparent defense mechanism that tries to maintain congruence between their flawed awareness and their sense of consciousness.

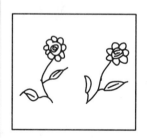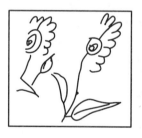

This figure shows how subtle and complex the deficit can be. A hemineglect patient was asked to draw a copy of two normal flowers (*on the left*) with the prototype visible all of the time the drawing was being made. The box on the right shows the result. Note that the patient did not simply ignore the flower on the left and draw only the one on the right. Instead, the left part of each flower was ignored and the right side was drawn with exaggerated detail.

An even more bizarre neglect effect is illustrated by a story recounted by a physician-researcher regarding a patient who had a stroke that resulted in left-side neglect. A nurse found the patient on the floor and helped him back into bed. After this happened again, the doctor arrived and asked the patient what the problem was. The patient replied, referring to his neglected left arm, "There's an extra arm in my bed and I keep trying to throw it out." A strange malady indeed!

MOTOR PATTERNS

Motor patterns, not individual muscle movements, are coded in motor memory, reflecting the fact that there is more than one way to make a set of movements that achieve the same result. For example, here are two versions of my first name as I write it in my usual signature.

The top sample was signed with a pen. The bottom one (adjusted to be the same size) was originally tens of times larger and was written with a piece of chalk on a blackboard. Writing with the pen mainly involved movements of my fingers and wrist. Writing with chalk on the board, my hand was fairly rigid and movements of my arm and shoulder were mostly responsible for the motor action. However, different as these two sets of movements were, involving almost entirely different muscles, the two signatures are remarkably similar.

This use of different output pathways is one example showing that learned motor memories are stored as plans and representations of the result of movements, and not simply as individual muscle movements that achieve them. This encoding is valuable because the same task may arise in different settings that require different body parts to accomplish it. Together, the combination of a plan in the cortical centers and the motion patterns that carry it out—derived primarily from the subcortical centers—accounts for the remarkable flexibility of our motor system.

Japanese Kanji characters illustrate just how pervasive motor components are in learning and memory. Each Kanji is like a "picture" that symbolizes a word (or words). For example, this one means "to think." (Interestingly, it is actually a combination of two others, the top half by itself meaning "head" and the lower half by itself meaning "heart.")

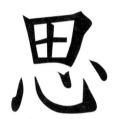

Japanese children learn about 2000 different Kanji symbols during their school years by doing calligraphy. A student first traces and then draws a Kanji over and over as the means of learning it. Further, the order in which each of the strokes is drawn is fixed and contributes to an individual Kanji's meaning. The motor nature of this learning leads to an interesting memory phenomenon. An English speaker trying to think of a word may say, "It's on the tip of my tongue." When a Japanese speaker tries to remember a Kanji, the person's hand is sometimes observed to unconsciously make calligraphic drawing movements. Or to put it another way, the Kanji is "on the tip of my finger."

WHEN DOES CONSCIOUSNESS SEE?

Everyone who has had a tennis lesson was taught to "watch the ball into the racquet" as opposed to looking at where the ball should go when it is hit. This advice makes sense; it is harder to hit something you are not looking at. And indeed, a good player will report seeing the impact. However, a simple calculation for a fast tennis serve reveals that the time it takes for the 100-mile-per-hour serve to cross the net and reach the receiver is less than the time it takes for the visual signal to get from the retina through the cortex. So, the ball is seen being hit after it actually is hit.

In fact, such delay is generally true. What we are aware of seeing always happened about 0.25 to 0.5 second ago because of the time it takes for the information to move through the nervous system. Our conscious "movie" of the world is time-delayed! Apparently, our consciousness is more a monitor of whether we accomplished our intent than the means of doing the action. So, why be consciously aware? One answer has to do with learning.

WATCHING, IMAGINING, AND DOING

Watching matters during learning. When we see someone else do a task, it gives us a pattern to try and follow. Recent research shows how individual "mirror" neurons may play a role in this process. Using the method of microelectrode recording, researchers found that there are premotor cortex cells in monkeys that fire when the monkey makes a particular hand movement and when the monkey watches the experimenter make the identical hand movement but not other movements.

Does the same process occur in humans? Well, newborn babies can imitate facial gestures just hours after birth. What kind of "mirror" processes might be involved? Neuroimaging studies in adults suggest an answer. A subject was instructed to move one finger in response to various signals or was instructed to only watch a finger being raised in a movie, without taking any action. In all cases fMRI showed activation of the same region in the premotor cortex. That is, a common subset of neurons is involved in seeing a task and in doing it.

Another neuroimaging study demonstrated that even imagination elicits appropriate motor activity. A subject was instructed to make a pattern of movements, touching adjacent fingers to the thumb in turn, or to just imagine doing so. Regions in the supplementary motor area, prefrontal cortex, and motor cortex were active when actual movement occurred. The latter two regions are known to be specifically involved in the motor output necessary for the movements but were not active when the movement was imagined. However, the same region of the supplementary motor area that was active in the actual task was also active during the imagined movement.

This result helps us to understand a phenomenon called *phantom-limb syndrome*. Many patients who lose an arm or leg report feeling sensations from the missing limb. These sensations are thought to be due to aberrant activity in the severed axons remaining in the stump or to an imbalance of activation in the remaining cortical circuitry. The sensation from the missing limb often subsides but sometimes turns into extreme pain that is hard to treat. The point is that cortical neurons that normally deal with the amputated limb are still functional, although they no longer receive appropriate inputs. This fact is best demonstrated by an fMRI study in which a patient was instructed to "move" the fingers at the end of his missing arm. As he tried to do so, the correct output area in motor cortex was activated, as if the fingers were still there.

To sum up, watching, imagining, and doing the same task all activate the same part of the brain in which the motor pattern for that task is stored.

CEREBELLUM

The cerebellum (from Latin, meaning "little brain") is a separate structure tucked below the cerebrum, dorsal to (behind) the brainstem. Its inputs and outputs communicate with other motor centers throughout the brain via tracts of fibers that make up the cerebellar peduncles.

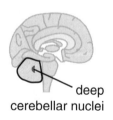

deep
cerebellar nuclei

The cerebellum's three main anatomic lobes reflect three major evolutionary stages. The oldest and most primitive vertebrates only have a flocculonodular lobe (synonym: *archicerebellum*), while primates have the largest posterior lobe (synonym: *neocerebellum*). In the next diagram these features are viewed looking at the front cerebellar surface.

All of the output from the cerebellum goes through the deep cerebellar nuclei, with one exception. The output of the flocculonodular lobe is via the brainstem vestibular nuclei, which are homologs of the evolutionary newer deep nuclei. Cerebellar outputs terminate in numerous cortical and subcortical areas,

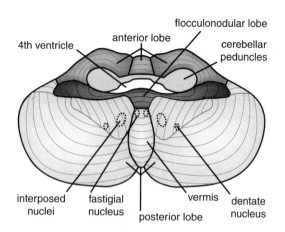

serving a wide variety of functions. Before these are described, it is useful to understand the local neuronal interactions that underlie all of cerebellar function.

THE PURKINJE CELL CIRCUIT

The *Purkinje cell*, introduced in Lecture 1, is the focal point of all cerebellar circuitry, as shown in this diagram (in which the cell on page 4 is reproduced in oblique view). Recall that the Purkinje cell's dendritic field is extremely dense but lies in a thin plane. The

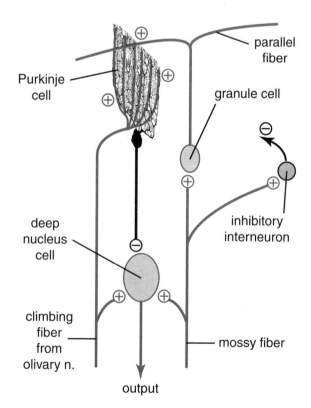

dendrites receive two major types of excitatory inputs. Every Purkinje cell is innervated densely and directly by one climbing fiber that comes from the inferior olivary nucleus of the brainstem. This nucleus integrates information from many motor centers. Thus, its activity provides summary information related to many aspects of movement. The second type of excitatory input is indirect, from a special class of cells called *granule cells* that receive input from mossy fibers. The granule cells give rise to a system known as parallel fibers that synapse with a large number of Purkinje cells that lie along their projections. Because mossy fibers originate in specific brainstem nuclei, this input is somewhat more focused than that of the climbing fibers.

It is important to note that the output cells of the cerebellum in the deep nuclei also receive excitatory input from the climbing and mossy fibers. The other input to these cells comes from the axons of the Purkinje cells and is inhibitory. This circuitry is best understood as follows.

Purkinje cells, besides their excitatory inputs, also receive numerous inhibitory inputs from cerebellar inhibitory interneurons. Together with the excitation, the inhibition contributes to each Purkinje cell being a summation point for motor-related information. This information is sent to neurons of the deep cerebellar nuclei. Those same cells also receive a slightly different excitatory picture from the same inputs that drive the Purkinje cells. But, because the Purkinje cell input to these deep nucleus cells is inhibitory, the cells are acting like little comparison machines. That is, excitation can be thought of as addition and inhibition as subtraction, with the result being action potentials if the excitation prevails. What is being compared is the excitation that is reaching the cerebellum, with the complex analysis of that same information by the Purkinje cell circuitry.

We can see this comparison in action by using a somewhat idealized example. Imagine that a cell in one of the deep nuclei is receiving information that a particular muscle in the left arm is supposed to be helping to move the arm at a certain speed in a specific direction. If the analysis carried out by the Purkinje cell indicates the movement is happening as expected, it signals strongly, thus providing strong inhibition to the deep nucleus cell. The inhibition cancels out the excitation and the neuron remains silent. However, if the Purkinje cell is not well activated—perhaps because the movement is not going as expected—the deep nucleus neuron will receive some excitation, causing it to fire action potentials that are directed to specific muscles in a way that helps to correct the movement. Thus, the Purkinje cell circuit acts as a kind of quality-control monitor.

FUNCTIONAL ANATOMY

The organization of cerebellar circuitry mirrors its various functions. Therefore, examining the three major cerebellar subdivisions and their primary inputs and outputs is a useful way to understand cerebellar function. The phylogenetically oldest flocculonodular lobe is concerned primarily with balance and postural equilibrium. It monitors these conditions primarily via the vestibular apparatus of the inner ear. That apparatus projects its output to the vestibular nuclei, which then project to the flocculonodular lobe. This lobe also has a major role in coordinating eye movements with head movements, which is important for keeping the eyes steadily focused on a particular point while the head and body are moving. Not surprisingly, strokes

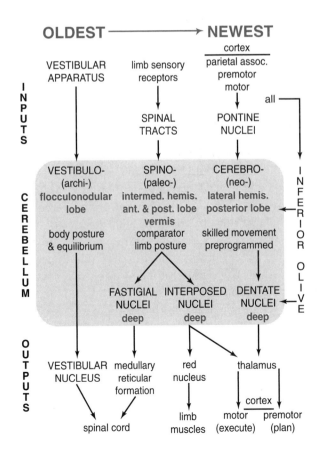

affecting this pathway lead to feelings of nausea and inability to balance properly.

The evolution of the spinocerebellar region (synonym: *paleocerebellum*) mirrors the evolution of limbs and the need not only to coordinate limb movement but also to do so with flexibility in response to various environmental features. Spinocerebellar inputs monitor how limb movement is progressing, and its outputs are organized to correct small deviations so that movements are smooth and accurate. People with lesions in this portion of the cerebellum start movements correctly but then carry them out in a jerky and ungainly manner, often overshooting the intended target.

The cerebrocerebellar region is composed of the intermediate lobe and vermis. It has evolved to the most complex elaboration in primates. It is associated with voluntary, skillful movements, like writing a signature or peeling a fruit. Its main inputs (via pontine nuclei) and outputs (via the thalamus) originate and end in the cerebral cortex. There the cerebrocerebellar area communicates with regions such as the premotor cortex that are involved in planning movement and with the motor cortex that executes movements via the pyramidal tracts. Reflecting the importance of skilled, voluntary movements to human behavior, 90% of all neurons of the deep cerebellar nuclei are in the dentate nucleus, the main output target of the neocerebellum.

BEYOND MOVEMENT CONTROL

The above analysis presents a picture of the cerebellum that would have been familiar 30 years ago, emphasizing it as a key component of the coordination of movement. Even the cerebellum's stereotyped neuronal circuitry is consistent with the idea of a computer-like controller that keeps movements on track. However, recent findings have shown that the cerebellum is much more important and interesting than this classic view implies.

A simple example shows a role for the cerebellum in identifying stimuli. A study used fMRI to show that sniffing the odor of vanilla caused activation of part of the posterior lateral cerebellar hemisphere (neocerebellum) in a concentration-dependent manner. This finding of specific olfactory responses in the cerebellum was not expected. Previously it was thought that such specificity resided only in the olfactory cortex.

However, the researchers suggested that processing such information in the cerebellum might be related to cerebellar output which provides feedback that can help to regulate the volume of a sniff based on the nature of what is being smelled.

Interlude—*Cerebellar Diseases*

• The ability of patients with cerebellar lesions to acquire what is known as a "classic conditioned response" was found to be impaired. Conditioned responses are the simplest form of learning, and thus this deficit highlights the role of the cerebellum in learning. Patients heard a tone and simultaneously had a puff of air applied to their corneas, causing a blink. After a number of trials, normal subjects who were presented with just the tone blinked without the puff of air. However, impaired individuals never came to associate the tone with the puff. That is, no conditioning could be observed.

• Studies using MRI found decreases in the volume of specific cerebellar regions of boys already diagnosed with ADHD. This finding led researchers to suggest that disruption of interactions between the cerebellum and prefrontal cortex may be involved in the loss of both motor control and higher-level functions that control behavior.

• Patients with cerebellar lesions were evaluated with standard neuropsychological tests of intellectual ability. They showed significant deficits in tasks that required the use of executive functions, such as choosing to initiate an action, and on memory tasks that required significant processing effort. Tasks that were relatively automatic were not impaired.

• Friedreich's ataxia and olivopontocerebellar atrophy and are inherited diseases that involve progressive impairment of motor pathways. Patients with both diseases were studied with tests of cognitive function that were not related to motor behavior. They were found to have measurable problems, apparently due to secondary effects of their diseases on cerebellar-cortical interactions.

• Study of patients with lesions in the posterior lobe of the cerebellum has led to the suggestion of a cerebellar "cognitive affective syndrome" characterized by symptoms such as impairment of working memory, planning, and abstract reasoning. These patients also demonstrated cognitive defects such as perseveration and difficulty with logical sequencing, as well as inappropriate affect.

COGNITION, LEARNING, AND MEMORY

The common thread of the clinical findings described in the Interlude is that the cerebellum is involved in much more than just the control of movement. One way to understand this expanded role is to realize that almost any aspect of thinking, learning, and remembering has a motor component at some time during its acquisition or subsequent associated behavior. With the use of neuroimaging techniques, researchers have been finding this "new" role for the cerebellum in normal individuals in a variety of situations. These results are summarized in the next figure adapted from a recent review article.

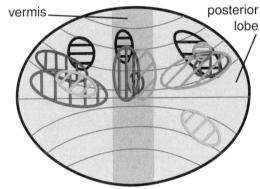

- ⓘ explicit memory retrieval
- ⊖ trajectory/ rotor pursuit learning
- ⊘ verbal working memory
- ⊖ classical conditioning
- ⓘ sequence learning
- ⊘ language/verbal working memory

A flattened view of part of the cerebellar posterior lobe and vermis is depicted here. The symbols show regions that were activated by various tasks. For example, verbal working memory for letters, words, and names utilized a strategy of silent, nonconscious rehearsal that involves some of the same parts of the brain as actually speaking these items. Studies showed activation of cerebellar regions that would normally be involved in the motor speech task, even though no actual speech occurred.

It is understandable that the cerebellum is involved when you learn a motor task, but the nature of its involvement is broader than would be expected based on classic views. That is, it is not simply the movements necessary for the learned task that involve cerebellar activity. Findings that the cerebellum is involved in retrieving explicit memories—words, events, or complex experiences that can be intentionally recalled—raise the question of whether and to what degree memory storage occurs there. Alternatively, cerebellar circuits could be involved in the search processes that retrieve memories stored elsewhere.

Further understanding of the varied roles the cerebellum might play comes from examination of the cortical targets that receive the output of the dentate nuclei. Initially, interaction between the cerebellum and motor cortex was understood based on the obvious role the cerebellum has in the coordination of movement. However, later studies demonstrated projections to the premotor cortex and the supplementary motor area, regions that are involved with planning of movements, not just with executing them.

It is probably the projections from the dentate nucleus to the prefrontal cortex (via the thalamus) that are the most surprising. The cerebellum contributes input to areas involved in higher functions of cognition and intellect such as planning, directing attention, and integrating emotion with behavior. These projections from the dentate nuclei are highly organized, with different dentate subregions mapping reliably to different cortical regions. Such organization suggests that something more is occurring than simply nonspecific modulation. What might this be?

A hint comes from an examination of normal humans trying to solve a difficult motor task. Subjects were given a puzzle-like problem that involved moving different colored pegs on a pegboard. With the use of fMRI, brain activation during the task was compared with activity that occurred during just simple movement of the pegs themselves. The puzzle task activated a region of the dentate nucleus that interacts with the part of the prefrontal cortical area involved in the planning of complex sequences of events.

Probably most surprising of all is the involvement of the cerebellum in mental illnesses such as schizophrenia and autism. Autopsies of autistic individuals have revealed losses of dentate nucleus neurons and Purkinje cells. Recent findings go well beyond even these diseases. Abnormalities in patients displaying psychotic behavior, extreme aggressive behavior, and inappropriate emotional responsiveness have been linked to cerebellar lesions.

As noted in the Interlude, a "cognitive affective syndrome" involving a general lowering of intellectual functioning can be discerned by generalizing these clinical findings. Recognition of such a condition has led to the suggestion of classifying cerebellar-based cognitive defects as "dysmetria of thought." Such a classification is parallel to the more typical involvement of the cerebellum in dysmetria. (*Dysmetria* is uncoordinated motor movement that misses its target.) The unifying idea here is (quoting Jeremy Schmahmann) that "the cerebellum detects, prevents and corrects mismatches between intended outcome and perceived outcome of the organism's interaction with the environment. In the same way as the cerebellum regulates the rate, force, rhythm, and accuracy of movements, so might it regulate the speed, consistency, and appropriateness of mental and cognitive processes."

In the end, the name "little" brain may not be an accurate one. The more we come to know about it, the more the cerebellum is coming to be recognized as a major partner in many brain functions.

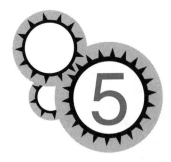

COMMUNICATING

REVIEW

Lecture 4 started by stressing that everything that anyone knows about you is due to your muscles. Thoughts are hidden, but movements—walking, talking, gesturing, writing—are the observable component of your behaviors. Some movements are voluntary and under conscious control, others are normally involuntary and don't require awareness, but all are controlled by hierarchical levels of processing and control in the spinal cord and the brain. Furthermore, parallel processing occurs in the brain regions responsible for these outputs just as in the brain regions dealing with sensory inputs.

Basic movement patterns are built into neural circuits within the spinal cord both as simple reflex arcs and as more complex central pattern generation circuits that have outputs initiating muscle contraction. These spinal circuits can operate in isolation, but are usually controlled by inputs from the brain. Lying just above the spinal cord, the brainstem contains localized centers that control and fine-tune movement. The extrapyramidal pathway is responsible mainly for posture and balance, while the pyramidal pathway that originates at cortical pyramidal cells coordinates fine, voluntary motor movements. Above the brainstem, the basal ganglia monitor and gate motor activity, allowing or inhibiting voluntary movements initiated in the motor cortex. The primary output areas of motor cortex interact with other cortical regions, such as those responsible for eye movements and areas of the parietal lobe that organize the sense of "self in space."

Neural circuits in motor cortex regions are the basis of outputs resulting from learned motor behaviors. However, the movements of very different sets of muscles can result in the same ultimate output. Thus "motor patterns" that correspond to an output result—such as a signature—are stored in the cortex, rather than specifications of individual muscle movements. Specific muscle movements result from the response of subcortical motor regions to motor-pattern signals that originate in the cortex.

An important recent finding shows that the same neurons responsible for *causing* motor movements are activated when these movements performed by others are *watched*, and even when the movements are imagined. This may be a basis of building specific memories, strengthening these memories, and recognizing the intent that underlies the movements of others.

The cerebellum compares intended motor movements with their actual occurrence, and then signals the ongoing corrections needed. It also serves as a site for memory storage of events that involve movement and monitors the appropriate output related to mental and cognitive processes.

"Mary said Joe left yesterday." Are you sure who did what? You might agree that "flying planes can be dangerous," but do we all agree how? These are examples of symbol-based communication and its complexity. If a few commas are added, "Mary, said Joe, left yesterday" probably means that it was Mary who left. Indeed, "flying planes" may be dangerous for a careless pilot, but a "flying plane" that falls out of the sky may be dangerous to people on the ground.

The ability for human communication to be as flexible and nuanced as it is depends on complex brain circuitry that no computer-based translation algorithm has come close to matching, which is why machine translations can be both crude and silly. We can barely explain how such complexity is organized in the brain. In large part this failure is because there is not a single, self-evident theory of language and its structure that we can map onto the structure of the brain. What we have are tantalizing hints from defects in language ability caused by strokes, brain lesions, and prenatal misdevelopment and from recent neuroimaging studies that try to capture and localize language in the brain as it happens.

This lecture introduces these hints and indicates the questions that need to be answered. It makes the point that once we get past regions of the brain responsible for direct input and output, the way we organize our understanding of brain structure is highly dependent on how we intellectually and culturally organize the structure of the world and our behaviors in it.

WHAT IS LANGUAGE?

Language is a collection of symbols that encode meaning. The word *meaning* implies cognition, that is, inner mental events that have intention and content beyond the action potentials that underlie their existence. Invoking such inner events is very different from conceptualizing the brain as a mindless behavioral device that processes inputs into outputs in a machine-like manner. In Lecture 9, we will have much more to say about this way of approaching the brain, but for now its importance is that we cannot try to understand how the brain makes language without understanding the intellectual nature of the linguistic process itself. For example, we need to know if language is a symbolic code that is entirely arbitrary or if it has underlying universals that occur in all language systems. If so, can we then find evidence for the basis of such universals in particular parts of the brain?

Interlude—*Anomia*

Anomia is the general term for the inability to name things. It is usually the result of a brain injury such as that caused by a stroke. What is remarkable is how specific the deficit can be. There are rare but interesting anomias that affect the ability to name animate things (e.g., horse) but not inanimate things

(e.g., car). Among the large variety there is color-name anomia and anomia for fruits and vegetables. The problem is not that the object is not recognized but rather that the word associated with it cannot be produced. For example, the person may say a word related to the object rather than try to name it. In fruit and vegetable anomia, the patient readily might say "pie" when shown an apple.

Another related deficit after a stroke is the loss of ability to use nouns but not verbs, or vice versa. It is not the word that is lost but its proper usage; the patient can use the identical word in one form but not the other. For example, the patient might be able to say, "The carpenter used a hammer," but not, "The carpenter needed to hammer in a nail."

Terminology note: *Anomia* is one of a large number of disorders of cognition that are often grouped into the categories of

    agnosia—disorder of recognition;
    aphasia—disorders of language; and
    apraxia—disorders of practice.

Appendix II contains a comprehensive list of these disorders.

When examined with MRI scans, damage from strokes associated with anomias is often found to be very localized. Also, similar anomias often affect approximately similar places in the temporal lobe from patient to patient. These similarities lead to the obvious hypothesis that some aspects of language may be organized into universal, content-specific modules in neighboring brain regions. In fact, Noam Chomsky forcefully presented this view.

Is such specificity really the case? Are anomias examples of disruption of certain innate features that are universal to all languages? This question of innateness is one of the major issues at the heart of this lecture. We have already seen a precedent for the idea in the visual system, where different parts of the visual cortex deal with color and motion. Now we are asking, are some aspects of language as innate and hardwired in the brain as are the functions in primary visual cortex?

To approach the question, we need to examine whether there are features common to all spoken languages. We start with listening and talking as opposed to reading, because the capacity for spoken and signed language seems to be innate. That is, children do not need to be explicitly taught to speak or understand what is said to them any more than they need to be taught to walk. This ease of learning is not true of reading, which requires many years of schooling.

LANGUAGE UNIVERSALS

The lowest common denominator of all spoken language is the fact that words are composed of a sequence of basic sounds called *phonemes*. Here are sound spectrograms of the syllables *di* and *du*. The individual phonemes /d/ (as in *d*ig), /i/ (as in h*ee*d), and /u/ (as in t*oo*) are indicated.

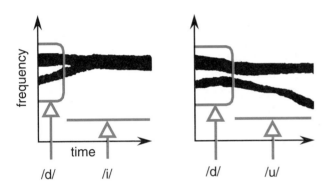

A spectrogram is a specialized recording of sounds being spoken. As usual, time progresses along the x-axis. The y-axis shows the intensity of the sound at each instant in terms of the frequencies from low to high that comprise it. The dark bands show the strongest frequencies. For example, the blue outline in each example highlights the most significant part of the frequency spectrum of the sound /d/. Note that it has two frequency bands of greatest intensity. In the left spectrogram these merge into a single band when the /i/ sound is made, but in the right spectrogram they diverge when the /u/ sound is spoken. In general, every phoneme has a somewhat different, stereotyped spectrogram (when normalized for voice pitch).

Linguists classify about 45 phonemes in English. Some languages have fewer and a few languages have more, up to about 150. Thus, even though phonemes are universal, any one element of the set may not be. Some sounds, corresponding to certain lip, mouth, and tongue configurations, are extremely common, probably mirroring both the basic sound-producing apparatus available to all human speakers and the neural circuitry responsible for the motor movements that make them.

The spectrogram makes a second point, namely, that even at the most basic phonemic level, things are not as simple as they seem. An English-speaking listener will hear the /d/ sound in *d*i and *d*u as identical, yet the spectrograms show they are somewhat different in the temporal course of their major frequencies. Why are the /d/ sounds heard as identical? They are because the way the brain processes even simple speech sounds is complex, and in part is based on our experience during language learning. The subtle frequency differences in the two /d/ sounds occur because of their interaction with the sound that follows them. However, we do not use these differences to convey different meanings in English. So, as adults we are no longer able to activate the neural circuitry needed to "hear" these differences. The same loss of discrimination is true in all languages. The /l/ sound (as in *l*ie) is not a phoneme in Japanese. A phoneme close to it is an "r-like" sound (unknown in English). Discrimination tests show that native Japanese speakers actually cannot hear the /l/ sound as different from their "r-like" sound. Their neural apparatus does not encode for it!

Lecture 8 on learning and memory will deal in great detail with this property of neural development called *plasticity*. For now, we can generalize to the following point. While there are probably some universals, it is hard to pin down exactly what, if anything, is innately invariant in language. Rather than a particular function itself being universal, it seems that particular brain locations have the ability to develop into local, module-like regions that can be used for language-like functions. As we will see later in this lecture, phonemes in all languages are "decoded" in approximately the same brain regions (near the temporoparietal cortical boundary), but obviously not identically.

PHONEMES AND WORDS

All languages distinguish between vowel and consonant sounds and have somewhat characteristic ways in which these sounds can be combined into syllables and words. For example, sonorance is an amplitude factor that tends to be greater at the peak of syllables than at their start or end, due to a buildup and decrease of airflow. Another constant of spoken language is that speech is inherently slurred. The boundaries between words are not always present as pauses, and there are inter-phoneme pauses that do not match word boundaries. This lack of pauses makes the task of learning to understand spoken language difficult in a way that is different from reading modern text, and thus all the more amazing.

Imaginelearningtoreadifallwritingwaslikethis.

Words differ among languages because there is no obvious relationship between the sound of a word and what the word signifies. Obviously, the development of related languages can be traced by examining common words, but across language groups variations can be extreme. Even onomatopoeic words (ones that imitate the sounds they are associated with) are more different than you might think, as this table shows for the words languages use for the sound a barking dog makes.

Arabic	haw haw
Danish	vov vov
Dutch	woef woef
English	woof woof
French	ouah ouah
Indonesian	gong gong
Japanese	wan wan
Russian	gav gav
Thai	hoang hoang
Ukrainian	haf haf

One common feature of all languages is the process of making new words from other words, either by adding a prefix or a suffix or both ("card" becomes "discarded") or by compounding ("mail" and "box" become "mailbox"). Compounding is a process that seems to reach an apex in German where such built-up words can be very long indeed, almost becoming sentences in themselves, such as *betriebsunterbrechungsversicherung*, a word that means "business-interruption-insurance." It is composed of the following parts:

betrieben, which means "to operate";
unterbrechung, "discontinuance" (itself derived from *unter*, "under" and *brechung*, "breaking"); and
versichern, "to insure."

SYNTAX AND SEMANTICS

The way that words go together in sentences comes under the headings of *syntax* and grammar, the structural rules that contribute to meaning. We are all familiar with the common English progression of subject (S), then verb (V), then object (O), which gives the sentence, "The car hit the tree" a different meaning from the sentence, "The tree hit the car," even though the words in both are identical. However, any one possible permutation of the S-V-O order can be found as the common way of phrasing in at least a few of the over 5000 known languages. So, it appears that the context that syntax provides is the commonality, but the exact form of the syntax differs from language to language.

Finally, in this brief study of what language is, we come to *semantics*, or meaning. We seem to have one or more "memory lexicons" where the sound of a word in its syntactic context is semantically related to meaning. These lexicons let the sound of "horse" call to mind a large four-legged animal that you can ride, and the sound conjunction "horse-around" mean something that usually does not involve such animals. This example returns us full circle to the anomias. Does the loss after a stroke of the ability to say "horse" when shown one, but to still be able to respond "horse-around" when seeing the appropriate picture imply multiple memory lexicons? If so, are they related? And, how do we "look words up" in these mental dictionaries? The speed with which we can retrieve words implies it is something other than the slow, serial process we employ when using a printed dictionary.

WHERE IN THE BRAIN IS LANGUAGE?

THE EARLY STUDIES

BROCA AND WERNICKE

Working in the 1800s, the French neurologist Paul Broca and the German neurologist Carl Wernicke generalized from observations of language impairment in their patients who had strokes and whose brains were later studied at autopsy. Broca observed that in patients who had no motor impairment but who had a loss of ability to speak (output), there was damage mainly in the posterior part of the inferior frontal gyrus (now called *Broca's area*). Thus, Broca and others suggested that frontal regions are involved in the planning and expression of language. Such disabilities are now called *Broca's aphasia*. *Wernicke's aphasia* is disruption of language comprehension (input) that involves damage in the posterior half of the superior temporal gyrus (called *Wernicke's area*). Later, *conduction aphasia*, which involves a disconnect between comprehension and speaking, was shown to involve disruptions of a major fiber tract, the arcuate fasciculus, which is one of the paths that interconnect these regions.

All of these aphasias were associated with lesions predominantly in the brain's left hemisphere. For almost 75 years following the work of Broca and Wernicke, researchers mainly studied patients with brain lesions that disrupted language—primarily because that is what was available—and such studies were the major basis for understanding brain and language.

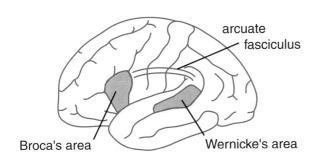

The regions shown as Broca's and Wernicke's areas in the figure are approximate, primarily because recent studies of hundreds of brains, using a large variety of techniques, have not yielded agreement on where the boundaries of these areas are. There is not even agreement as to what degree each is a single, discrete area with one function. What is agreed on is that every case of Wernicke's aphasia involves a lesion in the territory generally called Wernicke's area. However, the inverse is not true.

The lack of consensus probably has multiple causes, and exploring them is instructive in terms of trying to learn how the brain works. First, even though all adults have a brain of about the same weight and volume, the shape of their skull and thus the exact packing of the brain's sulci vary from person to person. Because comparative studies usually involve numerous

subjects, this natural variation in how the brain is folded makes it difficult to determine average parameters. Person-to-person variation is readily corrected when a region such as the primary visual cortex is studied, given the high exactitude of the basic retinotopic map and the precision of the techniques available for determining its localization. But, language is not regular in the way visual signals are, and thus the anatomic variations are hard to correct for.

Second, it is likely that Wernicke's and Broca's areas consist of numerous subregions. While every speaker of a given language may have the same subregions, it is not clear that the regions are identically arranged. For example, when and how language is acquired may lead to differences, as seen clearly when the brains of people who speak a second language are studied with fMRI. The areas of the brain that are active when a second language learned after age 7 is being comprehended often are different from those that are active when the native language is being comprehended. Regions within Wernicke's area that are active when the native language is listened to are inactive when the late-acquired language is heard. Further, the second language activates temporal and even frontal areas not normally responsive to listening to spoken language. In contrast, other studies showed that the later stages of processing of language, when meaning is most likely deduced, utilize many of the same regions of the brain as does all processing of a multilingual's languages, independent of when they were learned.

Third, careful study suggests that neither Broca's aphasia nor Wernicke's aphasia is a single syndrome. Use of a large bank of different tests of cognitive function usually can differentiate the symptoms of patients with the same initial diagnosis. The most striking result of such work has to do with reassessment of assigning only language production tasks to Broca's area. New studies with fMRI revealed that some parts of this area are activated when language comprehension occurs, a function classically thought to occur predominantly in and around Wernicke's area. An initial explanation of this finding was that silent, covert subvocalization was occurring as part of the comprehension. That is, in trying to understand the words being heard, the person was rehearsing the speaking of those words without being aware of doing so. Simultaneous activation of cerebellar pathways that might be involved in speaking strengthened this explanation, and it probably accounts for some of what is going on.

However, further study shows there is more to it, leading to a fourth category of causes.

It is hard to design a language task that uniquely distinguishes among cognitive categories, such as testing syntactic context versus semantics. Frontal activation in Broca's area during comprehension tasks is an informative example. It turns out that as a cognitive interpretative task becomes more difficult, more of Broca's area becomes activated. So, less activation occurs when trying to understand a sentence with two simple, consecutive clauses, such as

"The man drove away in his car that was red," than one with complex embedded clauses, like

"The man drove, on his day off, which was Thursday, with great care not to scratch the red paint, his new car."

This concept generalizes to most aspects of cognition; more difficult tasks usually involve larger networks of activation.

What conclusion can we draw from these many factors to help us as we look next at neuroimaging studies of language in the brain? Perhaps the safest thing to say is that language is processed via parallel pathways in a variety of brain structures, much like the other examples of parallel processing discussed in earlier lectures. Further, the more taxing the task, the more numerous are the parts of the language system that become involved. Finally, the way language is processed varies according to cultural and idiosyncratic factors.

Interlude—*Baby Talk*

The fact that language is culture-specific begins with the earliest usage of language in infancy. In the second half-year of life, babies start to babble, making what seem like bursts of nonsense sounds. However, careful study shows that the noises include *canonical babbling* sounds that are well-formed, consonant-vowel syllables that have adult-like acoustical features. The earliest syllables babbled are similar in all languages and seem to be determined mainly by the motor capabilities of the vocal cords, tongue, lips, and mouth. But by the age of only 9 months, the sounds start to be specific to the language that will ultimately be spoken. Babies raised in a bilingual environment appear to reflect both languages in their early utterances, and the

acquisition of two languages at once does not seem to hinder the speed at which each is acquired.

The early ability of babies to *hear* language-based differences in sounds is even more remarkable than their spoken production. There are various ways to determine if a newborn baby is paying more attention to one thing than to another. Using these techniques, a number of studies have shown that newborns attend more to speech in their native language than to similar talking in a foreign language. It is known that sounds can be heard in the womb and that the acoustic apparatus is functional in the last few prenatal months. Apparently this "hearing" begins to tune the child's language-perception neuronal circuitry even before birth. A related finding is that talking "baby talk" to a baby has a purpose, perhaps unbeknownst to the parent. When speaking to a baby, parents often talk in a voice pitch different from what they normally use. It turns out that the frequencies of baby talk match a baby's immature auditory pitch discrimination mechanisms very well.

NEUROIMAGING STUDIES

INITIAL SPEECH PERCEPTION

The easiest way to understand both the anatomy and the functionality of brain pathways that serve speech is to trace them from initial hearing to spoken output. In doing so, we will concentrate on the left hemisphere, the dominant speech hemisphere in most humans.

Signals that leave the cochlea reach the cortex by way of the complex, subcortical pathways discussed in Lecture 3. The first cortical region stimulated is the

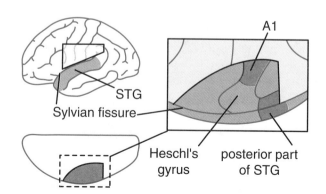

primary auditory cortex (A1), most of which is buried inside the sylvian fissure, as shown in the figure. The lateral and top views of the left hemisphere (*left side of figure*) show a wedge of cortex (*bounded by black outlines*) that is cut away so that the buried, superior surface of that region of the sylvian fissure can be seen (*viewed from above on the right*). The region on the superior inner surface of the temporal lobe where A1 lies is called *Heschl's gyrus*. From A1 the signal moves to adjacent A2, including a tonotopically organized area in the posterior portion of the superior temporal gyrus (STG). Although this initial analysis happens bilaterally, signals next converge predominantly onto left-hemisphere areas. Inputs from the right hemisphere project to the left side via the corpus callosum.

A1 and A2 are involved mainly in processing the frequency characteristics of language sounds as opposed to words themselves. Many of the next areas of interest lie adjacent to the sylvian fissure, giving rise to the shorthand designation that significant aspects of language are processed in "perisylvian cortex" (*peri-* means "around"). Following the signal through this region requires dissection of the various cognitive aspects of language.

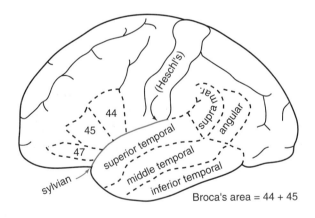

PHONEME DISCRIMINATION

The language signal spreads throughout Wernicke's area in the superior temporal gyrus, where further basic processing occurs. Phonemic discrimination is the next task, and a number of regions seem to be responsible. A major one is at the posterior edge of Wernicke's area at the temporoparietal border and in the angular gyrus.

Roughly simultaneously with phonemic discrimination, parts of the middle temporal gyrus and inferior temporal gyrus become activated. These parts are associated with object recognition and object naming, and the inferior temporal regions are exactly where anomia-causing strokes are localized. What is less clear is how this region and the phoneme regions interact.

WORDS, SYNTAX, AND SEMANTICS

Next, we must examine word recognition. Again, the exact role of the temporal areas is still unclear. However, it does seem that more of the angular gyrus gets involved, as do the supramarginal gyrus and some adjacent deep structures. That is, the analysis pathway is moving out of the temporal lobe toward the arcuate fasciculus and then to frontal regions, including Broca's area. This is the point where our current understanding clearly departs from the classic view. Recall that Broca's area was classically considered purely a language output region. Obviously, this hypothesis is no longer a tenable view. Not all of Broca's area is involved in the analysis; only the perisylvian regions of the anterior part (in Brodmann's area 45) are.

Word decoding is followed by understanding, which involves syntax and semantics. Although some syntactic processing accompanies word recognition in the posterior parietal regions, much of it is in the anterior perisylvian cortex. As amazing as it is that sounds are turned into words—that noise becomes information—the attribution of meaning to these sounds is perhaps the most astounding part of the process. It is in the anterior areas that mental lexicons are built and accessed.

There is evidence that syntactical and semantic aspects are processed in parallel circuitry. These aspects of language were distinguished in an fMRI study by a task that involved telling the difference between sentences in which either words (semantics) or clauses (syntax) were replaced by ones with similar or different meanings. Syntax was mainly localized to perisylvian regions of Brodmann's area 44, and semantics specifically activated perisylvian parts of area 47, anterior to Broca's area. However, this is not the entire story. Other prefrontal regions are also involved, as is a part of the anterior cingulate gyrus on the medial side of the hemisphere. What is the point of all this circuit tracing? It shows that there is indeed some correlation between the theoretical definitions of speech by linguists and the specialization of cortical areas for assessing distinct aspects of speech. It also shows there is a long way to go before we can suggest major functional pathways analogous to the "what" and "where" streams of visual information processing.

RIGHT HEMISPHERE AND PROSODY

What about the right hemisphere? It is activated by many of these same tasks, especially semantic ones. However, it has a relatively unique role when an entirely different aspect of language is considered, namely, *prosody*. "Don't talk to me in that tone of voice!" has been said to most of us at one time or another. What does tone have to do with what a word means? Tone evokes emotional qualities. Pitch, duration, and loudness carry meanings that we learn. They all are aspects of prosody. The lack of prosody is what makes machine language sound so artificial.

In English, a rising inflection at the end of a sentence usually indicates a question. For example, a rising inflection makes "You arrived yesterday?" into a question rather than a statement. However, although inflection use is universal, the meaning of any particular inflection is not. In some languages a falling inflection at the end of a sentence indicates a question. Another example of prosody, "twang" or "drawl," can let the listener guess where in the United States you might be from.

In some African and Southeast Asian tonal languages, pitch differences that are used when saying the "same" word give it entirely different meanings. For example, in Mandarin Chinese, "ba" said with a rising inflection means "to uproot," said in a flat midtone means "eight," and said with a falling tone at the outset and rising tone at the end means "to hold." It is interesting to note that such tonal language processing occurs in the left hemisphere, indicating its fundamental similarity to phonemic processing, which also occurs in the left hemisphere.

Analysis shows that while the prosody component of nontonal languages is not exclusively a right-hemisphere function, that side plays a predominant role. MEG has been used to observe localized brain activation, to show that while tonal information is swamped out in the left temporal areas by simultaneous noise, it is enhanced on the right side during such noise. PET neuroimaging has demonstrated that when the processing of changes in pitch occurs, right-hemispheric portions of Broca's area are activated. In studies of patients with an impaired right auditory cortex, pitch, timbre, and melodic discrimination were defective. However, pitch perception itself, via the normal left auditory cortex, was intact.

SPEAKING

Speaking starts with an idea. It must then be turned into semantically appropriate, proper syntax that then must be translated into motor movements. Thus, it is not surprising that the areas of the brain that are activated when the thought is being turned into a sentence to be spoken are much the same frontal regions as those used to understand speech. It is likely that the same mental lexicons are accessed, as are the perisylvian regions of Broca's area, especially in the posterior half (area 44). However, the activation of Broca's area now includes its more dorsal regions, superior to the perisylvian areas. Also, some activation even occurs in Wernicke's area. Next, activation moves into the supplementary motor area and then into cortical, motor output regions.

The failure of any part of the pathway can lead to speech deficits. *Dysarthria* is the name for any speech problem due to disruptions of the motor apparatus itself, especially the various muscles involved in speaking. Strokes can have effects that go beyond such simple mechanical difficulties. Strokes that affect the start of the speech process make it difficult to "find the right word," and those affecting the middle of the pathway can make sentences into jumbled "word soup." This deficit does not necessarily imply a defect in intellect. I once taught a woman with a Ph.D. in biochemistry whose speech was so distorted because of cortical misdevelopment that she often started a sentence in the middle and then said the starting words, or even started polysyllabic words with a middle syllable (e.g., sylla-poly-bic)!

Interlude—*Speaking and Signing: Language Is Language!*

American Sign Language (ASL) is used by deaf persons to communicate linguistically; it is a real language. The regions of the brain responsible for the production of hand signs were determined in a deaf, adult ASL user who did not otherwise have intelligible speech. The technique used involved stimulation with electrodes placed directly on the cortex. (The recording was done prior to surgery to localize areas that were causing epileptic-like seizures.) At the same time that the patient was instructed to make specific signs, cortical areas were focally stimulated. When part (area 44) of Broca's area in the left hemisphere was stimulated, the patient's ability to sign was degraded. His signs were "slurred" and words were confused. There were also signing defects when supramarginal gyrus (parietal) regions were stimulated.

What conclusions can we draw? It seems clear that areas involved in the production of language deal with making language happen, not just with making speech happen. In speaking, the muscle movements are facial. In ASL it is the hand doing the talking. Either way, many of the same language areas of the brain are responsible for the linguistic aspects of the task. This similarity may be related to the motor pattern generation of signatures discussed in the previous lecture. It also may be related to the origins of speech itself. The region in Broca's area stimulated in this patient appears to be homologous with an area of prefrontal cortex (F5) in monkeys that is responsible for hand movements.

READING

Reading and writing are culturally based events that arrived late on the evolutionary scale, being at most 10,000 years old. Thus, their invention occurred long after humanity was scattered throughout the world, and much too late for us to look for evolutionary changes in brain structure to explain reading and writing abilities. So, it should come as no surprise that when we examine reading, we find that it uses cortical regions that are already specialized for vision and language.

Reading involves recognizing individual marks as letters that comprise a word (orthography) as well as recognizing their meaning (semantics), part of speech (syntax), and perhaps their pronunciation (phonology). Obviously, reading is a visual task, and

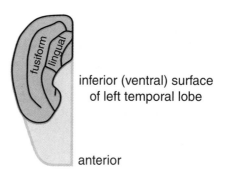

inferior (ventral) surface
of left temporal lobe

anterior

the early stages occur in visual cortical areas. Besides V1 and V2, which are activated by any visual stimulus, orthography seems to specifically activate deeper visual areas in the fusiform and lingual gyri, which lie on the inferior surface of the temporal lobe. After these areas have "turned" letters into words, further processing occurs in parallel. Some activation proceeds in the object-naming areas of the temporal cortex, the angular and supramarginal gyri become active, and there is specific activation in frontal cortical regions that we have already seen to be semantically important. Although both hemispheres are active, the left one predominates.

The complex nature of how all these regions interact to make meaning can be seen in the following example called the *Stroop effect*. It is named after the man who devised this task.

Black Blue

Subjects are shown words for color names such as these, with the words printed either in the same color as their meaning or in a color different from their meaning. The task is to name the color of the ink. Reaction time for saying the color is then determined. When the word and color do not match, the reaction time is longer than when the name and color are the same. Somehow the word information, which is very hard to ignore, interferes with the ability to identify the color when there is incongruence. This interaction is just one example showing that understanding language is part of a deeper cognitive system which is always working to make the myriad of inputs that are constantly bombarding us into something sensible.

Interlude—*Kana and Kanji*

Recall that the previous lecture presented Kanji characters as an example of the "tip of the finger" phenomenon. In Japanese there is a second writing system of alphabet-like characters called *Kana* that spells words just as in English. Interestingly, a Japanese adult can suffer a localized stroke that renders the person no longer able to read Kana but still able to read Kanji, or vice versa. This differentiation suggests that some aspects of Kanji/Kana reading may be localized in different brain areas. MRI has shown that such differences are indeed the case.

Reading Kana activates the same extrastriate and angular gyrus regions that reading English does. In contrast, reading Kanji characters preferentially activates a posterior portion of the inferior temporal gyrus, the same location that is activated when the task carried out is recognizing pictures of objects. That is, Kanji characters are treated initially by the brain as visual objects, not as letters.

FEELING

6

REVIEW

Lecture 5 dealt with overt communication between individuals based on language. Although language is a collection of arbitrary symbols that encode meaning, the way this symbolism is encoded in and enacted by the brain depends on specific cortical regions specialized for communication. Language universals include phonemes that are organized into words, syntax that governs the use of words and relation between words in sentences, and semantic meaning. Semantics—the relationship between the sound of a word and its meaning—is stored in specialized memory lexicons in cortical association areas.

Primary auditory areas process sound input into speech elements that then project to Wernicke's area, in the temporal lobe. Early studies of language distinguished Wernicke's area as the primary center of interpretation of language inputs, and a frontal lobe region (Broca's area) as the center that controls language output such as speech. However, more recent research shows that the two regions interact, and that each has some functions that overlap. Usually, language processing is located primarily in the left hemisphere, with the right hemisphere having a role in prosody, the tonal aspect of language. However, the right hemisphere homologs of Wernicke's and Broca's areas can take over primary responsibility for speech if the left hemisphere is damaged by accident or stroke.

It is important to recognize that language output can be more than sound. For example, signing used by the deaf is a legitimate language. Thus, it is not surprising that Broca's area organizes the motor outputs for sign language, as well as the motor outputs for spoken language. Put another way, language is a motor pattern that conveys meaning stored in mental lexicons, independent of the muscles moved. Reading starts in visual areas that decode the visual stimulus and then provide input to the mental lexicons used for language analysis.

Anger, guilt, sadness, hate, joy, nostalgia, mania, love, jealousy, surprise, fear, suspense, disgust, depression—these are words we use to describe our affective states. Are all of them emotions? How many different kinds of emotions are there? What is the difference between an emotion and a feeling? We know that emotions are essential to survival, but are they constructs that are learned or are they preprogrammed and hard wired in the brain? How can emotions, which are subjective states, be studied objectively? What do emotions have to do with memory? Why do we have emotions? Do animals have them?

You probably cannot easily answer all of these questions. This difficulty makes it hard to map these words into functions carried out by brain regions. It is like the issues we had mapping language onto the brain in the last lecture; we know there are puzzle pieces that may go together into a coherent picture, but we are not quite sure of the shape of each piece. We are not even sure whether particular pieces belong to the puzzle. And we certainly do not have all of the pieces yet.

This lecture deals with emotions and feelings. Together with the previous lecture, it starts a progression that moves from sensation and muscle movement to thought and mind. Not surprisingly, we will see that we know less about our higher functions than about the brain's basic inputs and outputs. In some cases our maps of understanding barely qualify as broad outlines, much like maps of the world in the 1500s. In this sense, the brain is the frontier of our times. Decades from now a lecture such as this one will seem quaint as new discoveries fill in embarrassing gaps in our knowledge.

EMOTION AND FEELING

DEFINITIONS

Before we can map the emotion-related centers of the nervous system, we need to know and understand what we are mapping. As with the problem we faced with language, we have a good idea about basics, but higher-order functions seem to be at the mercy of the theory we use to characterize and explain feelings and their functions. Progress will require interaction of psychological insight and neurologic investigation. The latter depends heavily on using modern, noninvasive neuroimaging techniques on normal individuals, as opposed to just studying the effects of strokes in humans or the results of brain lesions in animals.

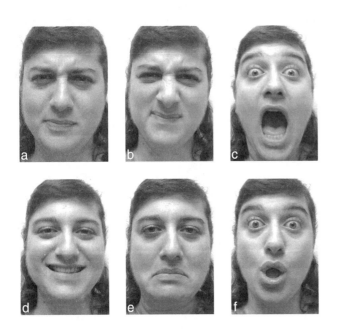

Let us start by looking at these pictures of human expressions that accompany emotions. Before reading further, can you tell the emotion that each one represents? Most adults can identify these (*from a to f*) as anger, disgust, fear, happiness, sadness, and surprise. These specific facial expressions occur spontaneously

in the presence of these emotions, even in people who are blind from birth. Perhaps more astounding, they are identical across all cultures: A happy face is a happy face, whatever the culture.

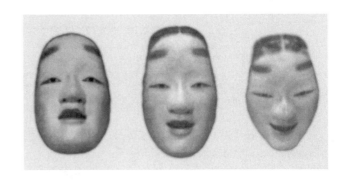

These pictures show a remarkable example of this universality and of our long-standing knowledge of the importance of facial expressions in social communication. In Japanese *Noh* Theater the actors wear wooden masks, such as this 350-year-old one. Obviously a mask cannot change expression. However, the remarkable thing about the masks is that they are purposely carved so that the viewer perceives different expressions if the wearer's head (and thus the mask) is tilted. The middle picture shows a neutral expression with the head not tilted. On the right, the head is tilted down 30° and the expression is clearly recognized as a happy one. In the picture on the left, the same mask is tilted 30° upward and expresses sadness.

The existence of universal, innate, spontaneous human expressions implies that they are prewired in our brains, not learned. Are these the only universal emotions? Well, there may be a bit of argument as to whether a few more should be included, but it is clear that the basic set is small. What about all the other words on the list at the start of this lecture? Some of them may be combinations of these basic emotions. Others, such as guilt, require us to define feelings.

An emotion has automatic, physiologic manifestations, including spontaneous facial expression, changes in blood flow to the skin, and a queasy stomach. For humans, there is also our conscious realization that an emotion is occurring, and the thoughts we then have about it. Antonio Damasio, a leading researcher, suggests the following distinction, which will be adopted in this lecture: The automatic, preconscious components, including the intrinsic physiologic sensations that accompany them, are labeled *emotions*. The conscious awareness that we have of emotions is labeled *feeling*. We know that we have both. We are also pretty sure that a cat has emotions, but we have no way of knowing whether or not it has feelings.

Feelings are complex because they involve conscious thoughts and interpretations that go well beyond the emotions that trigger them. For example, consider guilt. Most of us would probably agree it has components such as remorse, regret, and perhaps shame. At its core it involves a moral code, something that is cultural and learned. These are far different properties from the spontaneous response that characterizes a basic emotion. In short, guilt is a judgment, not an emotion.

Terminology note: A distinction between *emotion* and *mood* is often made. *Emotion* is a response to a direct stimulus that is present at the time. *Mood* is a more diffuse emotional state for which no immediate target is evident.

FUNCTIONS

Emotions and feelings are reliable guides that motivate action. If something feels good, like sex or tasting sugar, we are motivated to experience it again (*approach*). The reverse is true of fear, which will lead to *avoidance* behavior. There we have it: food, reproduction, and survival. Emotions are signals that trigger immediate behaviors related to these essentials. These are needs of all animals, and we will see that old parts of our brain are involved in the emotions associated with them.

The outward manifestations of emotion provide a reliable form of communication for social animals, especially primates. Such communication promotes survival of the group. It also leads to lying. The faces shown in the pictures at the start of the lecture are spontaneous responses to appropriate stimuli. The parts of the brain that control their occurrence are the basal ganglia and a few brainstem nuclei; there is no overt, higher cortical involvement. However, when we intentionally and voluntarily "make a face," the motor cortex takes over, provides the output that regulates the necessary muscles, and bypasses many of these lower centers. To all intents and purposes, the voluntary and spontaneous facial expressions look the same, but they are not. In a voluntary versus spontaneous smile, slightly different muscles are used, although the smile's recipient often overlooks the differences. So, although emotions may not lie, with a modern human cortex we have the ability to make facial gestures that are lies. Is this bad? That depends; sometimes tact is better than bluntness. Whatever else may be true, what cortical control does provide is the opportunity for a broader and more complex set of social interactions.

To understand the neural basis of emotions and feelings, we need to know how a stimulus leads to a physiologic response, how the response is automatically carried out, and how the cognitive overlay that we call a feeling is generated and interacts with emotions.

Interlude—*Sham Rage*

In a famous and important experiment done in the late 1920s, Phillip Bard reported a phenomenon he called *sham rage*. He surgically removed the entire cortex of a cat, as shown in the picture below, in which everything to the left of the blue line was excised. Upon awakening from anesthesia, the cat spontaneously exhibited a remarkable behavior pattern. It hissed, arched its back, bared its teeth, laid its ears back, and bristled its fur. This extreme, rage-like behavior was an exaggeration of what a normal cat might do when it is cornered or annoyed. Because there was no provocation, Bard used the word *sham* in his name for it.

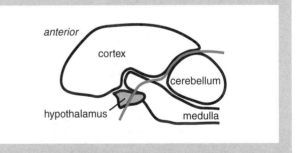

If you look closely at the figure, you can note a critical aspect of Bard's experiment. Namely, the posterior (caudal) portion of the hypothalamus was not removed. In fact, after removal of that region as well as the cortex, no sham rage occurred. These findings led to two important conclusions. First, emotion-related behaviors consist of complete, preprogrammed patterns, much like the "motor plans" discussed in Lecture 4. The occurrence of these plans is normally under cortical modulation, which was removed in the case of sham rage. Second, a trigger or organizer for the physiologic components of emotional behavior seems to reside in the hypothalamus. Further, the trigger does not require input from the cortex in order to be activated. Rather, the cortex keeps it in check. We will have much more to say about these important foundational principles of emotion and the brain throughout the rest of this lecture.

ANATOMIC OVERVIEW

This view of the medial surface of the left hemisphere summarizes the regions of the nervous system that have major roles in emotions and feelings. Most of them will be discussed in detail throughout the lecture and are introduced here.

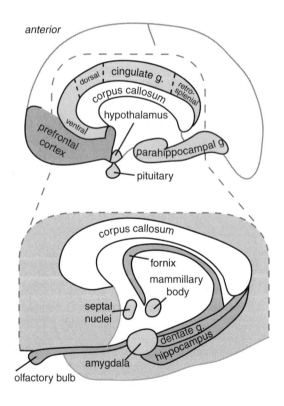

Broca was the first to propose what he called the *limbic lobe*, consisting of the gyri surrounding the edge (synonym: *limbus*) of the corpus callosum. In the

diagram, this is mainly the cingulate gyrus. However, he did not suggest functions for it. Others, using cytoarchitectonic criteria, added the cortical regions at the ventral edge of the ventricular space, mainly the parahippocampal and dentate gyri, to the limbic lobe. Subsequent work associated these regions with emotion, based on human behavioral deficits following strokes as well as animal lesion studies. Currently, we know that the cingulate gyrus has a clear role in processing feelings, as discussed further below. The exact role of the parahippocampal and dentate gyri in emotion is still unclear. (Their role in memory will be discussed in Lecture 8.)

Terminology note: Building on the name *limbic lobe*, scientists came to call this entire region the *limbic system*. Most of the regions discussed in this section are considered to be part of it. However, use of this name is decreasing, except as anatomic shorthand, because it does not accurately mirror the parts of the brain involved in emotion or for that matter, any single set of associated functions.

Other areas involved in emotion are the hypothalamus and a group of buried structures shown in the lower part of the figure, which is a cutaway diagram about one-third of the way in from the medial surface. The hippocampus is more involved in memory than emotion, so its discussion is put off until Lecture 8. The olfactory bulb and tract not only deal with odors but also provide the inputs that lead to the emotional connotations of smells. The amygdala is a central pivot point in the emotional circuitry of the brain. The septal nuclei and mammillary body are key stations along the emotion pathways, and the fornix carries many of the axons involved in those pathways. The most anterior area of the frontal cortex (called the *prefrontal cortex* to distinguish it from the more posterior areas of frontal lobe that are directly involved in motor control) interacts with many limbic structures to attribute meaning to emotional states.

Interlude—*The Triune Brain*

Paul McLean, an important neurologist of the mid-twentieth century who advanced our knowledge of the brain's functional neuroanatomy, proposed the concept of the *triune brain.* He suggested

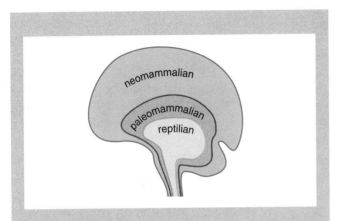

that three evolutionary levels could be seen in the primate brain in terms of both anatomy and function, sort of like a three-layered onion. The core is the reptilian brain (synonym: *archipallium*) that consists of the hindbrain, with a primitive cerebellum, and a midbrain. This brain reacts aggressively and automatically in the interests of self-preservation. The next layer is the *paleomammalian* brain. It includes the olfactory portions of the brain and, of interest to this lecture, much of the limbic system. Thus, with the evolution of this part of the brain emotion comes into play, making reactions more complex and varied than those of the reptilian brain. The most evolutionarily advanced layer, the *neomammalian* brain, comprises the bulk of the cortex and puts the emotion of the paleomammalian limbic system under the control of higher cognitive functions. However, the critical position of the emotional paleomammalian layer between the cortical brain and the rest of the body allows it at times to overrule, indeed to overwhelm, the more "thoughtful" newest brain.

It is not only the recognition and identity of functional evolutionary layers that make McLean's idea important. He also makes it clear that the brain's evolution is not simply a succession of increases in the size and complexity of small regions. Rather, wholly new parts came into being to serve expanded ranges of behavior, overlaying what was already there.

AUTONOMIC AND ENTERIC NERVOUS SYSTEMS

In this section we look at the automatic, physiologic manifestations of emotion, the patterns of

response that are "built in." The parts of the brain involved include the sympathetic, parasympathetic, and enteric systems, and the hypothalamic and brainstem regions that coordinate their functions.

SYMPATHETIC AND PARASYMPATHETIC SYSTEMS

ANATOMY

The sympathetic and parasympathetic systems comprise the autonomic system and usually control functions in opposite directions. For example, parasympathetic action slows the heart rate and sympathetic activation speeds it up.

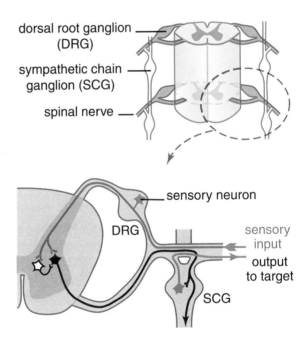

Sympathetic output is illustrated in this figure. Axons of its output neurons leave the spinal cord in the thoracic and upper lumbar segments of the spinal cord. These output axons project only a short way from the spinal cord to a sympathetic chain ganglion. There, most synapse with a final output neuron whose axon travels long distances to its target. Others (*not shown here*) pass through the chain ganglion to another ganglion nearer the target, before synapsing. In either case the final output neuron uses norepinephrine (synonym: *noradrenaline*) as its transmitter to the target tissue. Note that the output neuron in the spinal cord also projects, via the sympathetic chain, to ganglia above and below its own segment. This projection allows an integration of regional outputs. Finally, the target tissues return signals to the spinal cord that provide feedback to assist in homeostasis. Note that the soma of these sensory neurons is in the dorsal root ganglion.

The output neurons of the parasympathetic system follow a different pattern. They lie in the brainstem, in the uppermost (cervical) section of the spinal cord, and in its lowest (lumbar and sacral) sections. Every parasympathetic output neuron has a relatively long axon that terminates near its final target, where it synapses onto another neuron in a localized region called a *ganglion*. That ganglionic neuron then sends its axon to the target, such as a muscle of the iris of the eye, a salivary gland, the heart, or the lower bowel. There it releases the neurotransmitter acetylcholine.

PHYSIOLOGY

The sympathetic system gets the body ready for action, such as fighting or fleeing. To do so, it can activate its various targets simultaneously. This activation causes an increase in heart rate, dilation of blood vessels to the muscles and brain, a decrease in blood flow to the viscera and skin, a decrease in digestion rate and closing of sphincters, sweating, an increase in blood glucose levels, and dilation of the pupils. These responses are enhanced by the simultaneous release of norepinephrine into the bloodstream, which also travels, more slowly, to appropriate target organs. Concerted activation of the sympathetic system turns down activities not needed for immediate action and assists other organ systems, especially striated muscles, to function optimally. This sympathetic response is the physiologic accompaniment to strong emotional responses

In contrast to the sympathetic system, the parasympathetic system is not set up to cause a set of quick actions. One way to see why is to realize that its outputs generate activity that is opposite to that of the sympathetic pattern. Look back at that pattern, invert each action, and you'll see that the result would be both dysfunctional and messy. Instead of instant mass action, the parasympathetic system is set up to provide a body maintenance role, more like "rest and digest" than "fight or flight." For example, it promotes

digestion and the storage of fat and glycogen, increasing energy reserves.

It is important to realize that from moment to moment you usually are not either fighting or resting but are going about a wide range of daily activities. To accomplish this, the sympathetic and parasympathetic systems are always "on" to some extent, maintaining the metabolic balance in your organs that is necessary for living. Put another way, the two systems provide the complementary actions necessary for homeostatic balance in the body. As well, the sympathetic system can assume its immediate fight-or-flight role when needed.

Interlude—*Cranial Nerves*

In the discussion of the parasympathetic system, we mentioned the fact that much of its output originates in the upper cervical region of the spine and in the brainstem. Some of that output is via cranial nerves. The cranial nerves are too important to skip over, so they get their own Interlude and an appendix. Most of them are responsible for much more than autonomic functions. For example, some innervate the muscles and sense organs of the head and face. Both outputs to those targets and inputs from them are carried in the cranial nerves. There are 12 such nerves and their functions are described in Appendix III. One of the banes of the life of anatomy students is the need to memorize their names and corresponding number. For this purpose many mnemonics have been devised, with the first letter of each word being the first letter of the name of a cranial nerve, in numerical order. One of these that can be repeated in polite company is, "On Old Olympus Towering Tops, A Finn And German Viewed Some Hops." Look in Appendix III to see what this mnemonic stands for.

ENTERIC NERVOUS SYSTEM

The enteric nervous system is probably the body's best-kept neuronal secret. Most of us are unaware that built right into our "gut" is a vast network of neurons that organize all of its digestive-related movements. This anonymity is even more surprising because the enteric nervous system has more neurons than the entire spinal cord! When it works well, we are not aware it is there; when it does not work, we can barely attend to anything else but the pain or discomfort in our belly or the results of malfunctioning intestines. The enteric system is the "gut feelings" system that is a major component of the physiologic aspect of emotion. The enteric nervous system receives inputs from the rest of the nervous system; however, it is able to function entirely on its own.

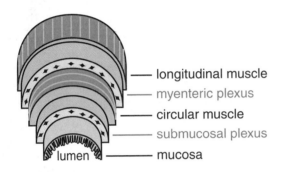

— longitudinal muscle
— myenteric plexus
— circular muscle
— submucosal plexus
lumen — mucosa

The figure shows a partial cross section of the intestine, cut away to reveal the major layers of the enteric system. Adjacent to the actual intestinal mucosa, the submucosal neuronal plexus plays the main role in controlling the secretory functions of the gut. As well, it contains sensory neurons that provide feedback related to what is happening and what is needed. It is surrounded by the layer of circular muscle. Over the circular muscle lies the myenteric neuronal plexus, the major source of motor neurons that innervate gut muscle, including the outermost longitudinal muscle layer.

The point of all this structure is best captured by one of its foremost researchers, Michael Gershon, who writes in his book *The Second Brain*: "A great deal of highly sophisticated chemistry has to take place to liberate what we need from what we eat. . . . To get the necessary chemical reactions to proceed, the environment within the bowel has to be regulated, the contents of the gut have to be mixed, and the enzymes that attack foods have to be present in precisely the right concentrations. . . . It is necessary to have a system of sensors in place that can detect the progress . . . on a moment-to-moment basis. The information . . . then has to be coordinated to assure that the internal environment within the gut will favor digestion and absorption. . . . It makes good sense for evolution to have put the requisite brain right in the organ itself." **Neuronal**

inputs from outside the enteric system innervate both plexus layers to provide influences from the rest of the nervous system that can modulate all of this activity.

Interlude—*Loss of Gut Feelings*

G. W. Hohmann carried out a remarkable study in the 1960s of ex-soldiers with spinal cord injuries. He correlated the site of the damage with the person's ability to report his own feelings of fear and anger. The result was that the higher the lesion in the spinal cord (cutting off greater amounts of visceral sensation), the less able the individual was to report the nature of his emotions.

Antonio Damasio reported the results of studying patients with lesions of the prefrontal cortex associated with emotion. These patients simultaneously lost the ability to sense their emotions in situations that involved risk and conflict, and the ability to decide rationally how to deal with such situations. That is, their emotions were disconnected from their feelings and cognition. He explained the disconnection by proposing the somatic-marker hypothesis, saying, "[I suggest] that the delicate mechanism of reasoning is no longer affected, nonconsciously and even on occasion consciously, by signals hailing from the neural machinery that underlies emotion." That is, gut-related signals are necessary somatic markers of emotion that are sent to, recognized, and acted on by areas in the prefrontal cortex. Both this theory and the work of Hohmann show how our rational abilities and our emotions are inextricably interlinked.

HYPOTHALAMUS AND BRAINSTEM

In this section we will examine how brainstem centers and the hypothalamus interact with and modulate the activity of the sympathetic, parasympathetic, and enteric systems.

ANATOMY OF THE HYPOTHALAMUS

The hypothalamus is the brain's master controller of the body's autonomic and endocrine activity.

Its endocrine control function is based on its communication with the pituitary gland, which lies immediately below it. The pituitary, in turn, releases a large variety of hormones and hormonal control molecules into the bloodstream, which carries them to neuronal (and non-neuronal) targets throughout the body.

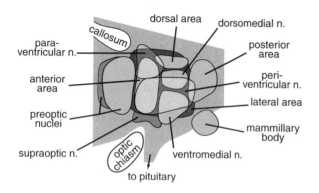

The hypothalamus is not a unitary structure but is made up of numerous tightly packed, interrelated nuclei. Besides the nuclei that affect the pituitary, there are ones that provide neural output to the autonomic and enteric systems. More to the point of this lecture, many hypothalamic nuclei receive emotion-related inputs from the limbic system. The picture shows the various nuclei that comprise the hypothalamus, looked at from the medial surface (i.e., the lateral area is farthest away and anterior is to the left). Refer to the picture earlier in the lecture to get a sense of the position of the entire hypothalamus relative to the rest of the brain.

The hypothalamus is a bilateral structure, and only its left-hemisphere components are shown in the figure. A mirror set of nuclei exist in both the right and left hemispheres. Presently, we have little knowledge of a difference, if any, in function served by a given nucleus in the right hemisphere versus its homolog in the left hemisphere.

Interlude—*Bilateral Symmetry*

You have duplicates of many anatomic structures such as two arms, two legs, and two kidneys because vertebrates are bilaterally symmetric. In the cortex, bilateral symmetry is reflected in the fact that most cortical structures exist as pairs, with one member in each hemisphere. It is easy to understand this duplication when sensory areas are considered. For example, the right primary visual cortex, area 17, is mirrored by left-hemisphere area 17. Their difference only involves which part of the visual field they "look at." Similarly, considering basic motor outputs, it is easy to understand the fact that the right motor cortex controls the left side of the body, and the left motor cortex controls the right side.

When we get to higher functions such as speaking, emotions, feelings, and thinking, the situation is not as simple. For example, Broca's area in the left hemisphere is involved in language production, but its mirror-image area on the right side is not significantly involved. We are not yet sure exactly what the functions of the region on that side are, although it appears to play some subtle role in expressing meaning. Similar uncertainty extends to many of the "higher" areas discussed in this and the following lectures. However, it is probably safe to say that such regions are not redundant, and that they do not serve as spare backups held in reserve. Rather, the few hints we do have suggest specialization for different aspects or features of the same function (e.g., different types of emotions may be served by one hemisphere or the other).

PHYSIOLOGY

The following, highly simplified diagram depicts some of the interactions of the hypothalamus, brainstem nuclei, and the limbic areas that are the most relevant to the physiologic aspects of emotion.

• The limbic structures can exert significant control over the autonomic and enteric systems via limbic input to most of the hypothalamic nuclei.

• The nucleus of the solitary tract in the medulla is a focal point, serving as a main recipient of sensory inputs from the cardiovascular and gastrointestinal systems, as well as signals from the hypothalamus that modulate these inputs. It distributes the results of these interactions to other brainstem nuclei, the hypothalamus, and cortical limbic areas.

• The three nuclei in the shaded area at the bottom of the figure provide output to the autonomic and enteric systems, especially via the vagus nerve.

We can get a good idea of how the physiology of emotions is controlled by following an incident from

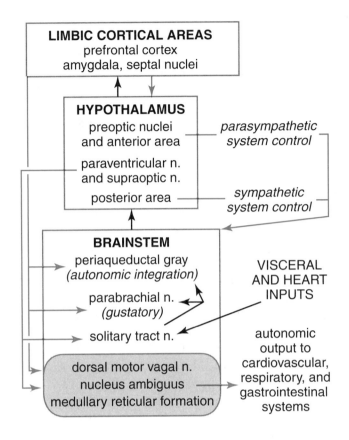

LIMBIC CORTICAL AREAS
prefrontal cortex
amygdala, septal nuclei

HYPOTHALAMUS
preoptic nuclei
and anterior area

*parasympathetic
system control*

paraventricular n.
and supraoptic n.

posterior area

*sympathetic
system control*

BRAINSTEM
periaqueductal gray
(autonomic integration)

parabrachial n.
(gustatory)

solitary tract n.

VISCERAL
AND HEART
INPUTS

dorsal motor vagal n.
nucleus ambiguus
medullary reticular formation

autonomic
output to
cardiovascular,
respiratory, and
gastrointestinal
systems

start to end. Start by realizing that any change in the world around you can precede danger or opportunity or a need for action. So, the brain is especially tuned to sense changes.

Imagine you are lying in bed, falling asleep at night, vaguely attuned to the constant and familiar sounds of your house. Then, a new sound occurs. It is not loud but it is different—a change from the ongoing noises. Your body goes on alert even before you are aware you heard the noise, triggering evolutionarily old systems that prepare for action. This alerting happens because the signal moves from your auditory system to limbic regions that are especially responsive to newness and difference. Those structures send signals to the posterior area of the hypothalamus, which in turn starts to activate the sympathetic nervous system, the "fight-or-flight" machinery, preparing for action.

The signals move to the dorsal motor vagal nucleus and the medullary reticular formation, which in turn pass the activation on to your heart and your gut. The heart responds by suddenly increasing its rate, and the intestines flutter as their motor activity is briefly inhibited. This all happens so quickly that you are not yet aware you heard something strange. What

you first become aware of is your change in heart rate and the "butterflies" in your gut, because sensory neurons in the viscera send signals of those physiologic changes back up the spinal cord to the solitary tract nucleus in the brainstem. The solitary tract nucleus signals other brainstem areas, calling them into action. More important, these signals also reach your cortex. Some of them go to the amygdala, the region that initiates fear. Others go through the thalamus to somatosensory regions. Suddenly you are physically aware of your physiologic changes and have associated a negative fearfulness with them. Realize that this is the first moment that emotion has become feeling, and is the first alert to your conscious self that "something is happening." That is, what you are responding to is not the sound, nor the output of the sympathetic system, but rather the signal coming back from your gut.

Now you are alert and your short-term memory recalls the sound that started this all, or at least sensitizes your hearing to be more acute. There the noise is again! But now your cognitive, conscious self has been brought into the picture. You tense up, sending more signals to the hypothalamus from the cortex and amygdala, getting the sympathetic system even more active. Meanwhile you think quickly: Is the noise the cat or a cat burglar? A moment of thoughtful analysis recalls that you forgot to let the cat in. Fear turns to annoyance and the sympathetic system settles down, even though you have to get up and go let the beast in.

CORTEX

In this section we look at the apparatus that turns emotion into feeling, concentrating first on a key structure in this drama, the amygdala. It is important to emphasize that all of the cortical areas related to emotion and feeling function in parallel; there is no single "seat of the emotions." The details of this parallel processing are not yet well understood, but it occurs here just as it does in the various sensory systems.

AMYGDALA

Amygdala comes from a Latin word meaning "almond" and roughly describes the shape of this region as envisioned by early anatomists. It is pictured

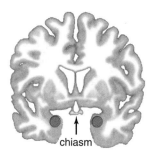

chiasm

in the diagram at the start of the lecture and depicted here as the bilateral, circular blue regions in a coronal section of the brain. The presence of the optic chiasm indicates that this is a relatively anterior section, showing you that the two amygdalae are buried near the front of the temporal cortex.

Like the hypothalamus, the amygdala is more of an anatomic definition than a single functional structure. It is composed of at least three subregions that have different roles. However, characterizations are hard to make because of its small size. It is likely that higher-resolution MRI studies made with stronger magnets will clarify this issue.

One thing that is clear from fMRI studies is that when the feeling of fear occurs, the amygdala is active. Fear is the predominant emotion that the amygdala is involved with, while related feelings such as anxiety activate other limbic areas in the striate nuclei. A demonstration of the role of such fear inputs is that patients with extensive, bilateral amygdalar damage do not experience fear. They also are unable to judge whether a picture of another person indicates if they are trustworthy or not. Further, it is not possible to produce conditioned responses based on negative emotional stimuli in such patients. It is also hard for them to form factual memories that have emotional content. In normal individuals, the amygdala is important in forming memories associated with both positive and negative emotions, particularly through its interconnections with the hippocampus.

The amygdala becomes active even if you only read words that have threatening connotations. It is also active in situations involving reward and punishment. In one interesting study, subjects played a game involving winning (reward) or losing (punishment) while simultaneously being scanned with brain imaging techniques. The left amygdala specifically activated when winning was the outcome, and the right amygdala was activated by losing.

There is significant interaction between cognitive functions such as reasoning and the fear-driven activity of the amygdala. For example, looking at faces that elicit a fear reaction is an especially potent stimulus. However, when a person is asked to simultaneously perform a distracting cognitive task, such as identifying the age and gender of the face, activation of the amygdala is inhibited.

ODOR AND EMOTION

Odor-sensing receptors in the nose send their axons to the olfactory bulb, which then provides inputs directly to cortical and limbic regions via the olfactory tract. In this way, smell differs from the other senses, which must pass their information through the thalamus on the way to the cortex. Such direct input reflects the evolutionary origin of these pathways in the old "reptilian brain." The relatively direct input of odor information to the hippocampus, which is involved in memory formation, is probably why smells can evoke vivid memories. Most of us are familiar with the experience of a smell, perhaps damp leaves in autumn, bringing up an entire scene from some special moment. Odors also can have strong emotional connotations. Negative ones are in part mediated by the amygdala because signals representing unpleasant odors are channeled directly to it via the olfactory tract.

The role of odor information in memory formation by the hippocampus can have startling, unintended consequences. In one study, children were asked to perform a particularly difficult and frustrating task. Simultaneously, an odor, neither particularly pleasant nor unpleasant, was purposely introduced into the room. The children did not report being aware of the odor. Later, they were separated into two groups. Each group returned to the room and was asked to carry out a new, hard, but accomplishable task. For one group there was no odor, and for the other the previous odor was again present. Those who worked in the presence of the odor did not perform as well as the children in the other group. Nonconsciously, they associated the odor with frustration and failure, thus giving up before solving the new problem. This finding is supported by many other studies. For example, people report that their mood is improved by the presence of a faint, pleasant odor of which they are not consciously aware until it is called to their attention.

CINGULATE GYRUS

There is extensive involvement of prefrontal cortical areas in determining the nature and immediate importance of emotional experience and in deciding on an action that is to be taken in response. Much of this function involves directing attention as well as accessing memory to compare present with past. First, the cingulate gyrus is our area of focus. Then, other prefrontal regions are discussed.

Refer back to the figure on page 60 and note that the cingulate gyrus is a rather extensive structure that essentially "covers" the corpus callosum. If you look at the diagram of Brodmann's areas in Appendix I, you will see this gyrus is subdivided anatomically into at least eight areas. So, it should come as no surprise that many different functions occur here. The single common feature of the gyrus is its close correspondence to the middle level of McLean's triune brain concept.

Three of its regions, labeled *ventral*, *dorsal*, and *retrosplenial* in the diagram on page 61, are especially relevant to this lecture. The ventral and dorsal regions comprise an area commonly called the *anterior cingulate cortex* (ACC), a part of the prefrontal cortex. They are grouped together because both have interconnections with other limbic regions and are activated during tasks that require a high degree of mental effort.

The dorsal region of the ACC is involved in memory and attention and is discussed in the following two lectures. The ventral region is highly interconnected with the amygdala, striate nuclei, hypothalamus, and limbic brainstem nuclei. Its major roles seem to be assessing the relevance and importance of emotional information and helping to regulate emotional responses via outputs to the autonomic, enteric, and endocrine systems. The ventral ACC is active when subjects pay attention to their emotions and in situations evoking sadness, anxiety, and phobias.

Interlude—*Stroop Revisited*

A Stroop effect–type experiment was used to demonstrate the different functions of the dorsal and ventral ACC. Subjects were shown a word that was displayed three or four times, but only once per line, as in the following examples.

The task was to report how many lines were present. Subjects were instructed not to pay attention

house	three	
house	three	murder
house	three	murder
house	three	murder

to the words but instead to try to respond as quickly as possible. A set of words such as *house* was a neutral control. In one set of trials the word *three* or the word *four* was displayed, in some cases three times and in other cases four times. When the word *four* was shown three times, it produced a dissonance condition similar to showing the word *black* printed in blue ink, discussed in Lecture 5. During such dissonance conditions, the dorsal ACC was especially active, indicative of its role in helping to make decisions about cognitive information under confusing conditions. When an emotionally charged word such as *murder* was used in the experimental trial, the ventral ACC was active. It was dealing with the emotional content of the presentation, even though that content had nothing specific to do with the task.

In related experiments, the emotional and cognitive regions interacted reciprocally. During very demanding cognitive tasks, the ventral ACC actually became deactivated while the dorsal ACC became highly active. The reverse occurred during highly emotionally charged tasks. This example shows how emotions and "rational" cognition can interfere with each other.

The ventral two-thirds of the posterior region of the cingulate gyrus is called the *retrosplenial area* because it surrounds the back curve of the callosum, called its *splenium*. The region has been recognized only recently as having a major role in emotions. Anatomically it connects extensively with the prefrontal cortex, including the anterior cingulate gyrus, the parahippocampal gyrus, as well as other cortical areas. The retrosplenial region plays a role in evaluating emotionally charged sensory stimuli, independent of whether action is taken in response to them. Similar to the ventral ACC, it is inactivated during intense cognitive tasks, again emphasizing how emotion and cognition seem to compete with each other.

OVERVIEW OF PREFRONTAL AREA

The prefrontal cortex is functionally and anatomically divided into three regions, the dorsolateral area (discussed in the next lecture) and the ventromedial and orbitofrontal areas. Prefrontal functions overlap and interact. Because we do not yet fully understand the functional richness of this part of the brain, the descriptions that follow are oversimplified.

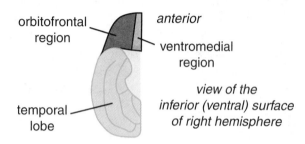

VENTROMEDIAL REGION

The ventromedial region integrates and initiates patterns of emotional behavior. Some evidence suggests that this region is where emotional memories are stored and that these memories may be activated as part of the "somatic marker" events that Damasio postulated. Patients with lesions in this area fail to demonstrate normal emotional arousal. For example, when shown sexually arousing pictures or ones that normally cause fright or disgust, they do not respond any differently than they do to placid scenes. Such patients are often described by their acquaintances as having "flat personalities" and "lacking emotion." Also, because of their inability to monitor emotions in others, they often behave in socially inappropriate ways and use obscene speech without any hesitation, seemingly oblivious to normal moral standards. In sum, at least one group of functions of the prefrontal ventromedial area is to elicit emotional memory and use it to generate emotional responses and to interact in socially appropriate ways.

ORBITOFRONTAL REGION

The orbitofrontal region seems specialized for a somewhat different but overlapping set of emotionally related functions. Its malfunction is implicated in obsessive-compulsive disorder (OCD). The major inputs to the region are olfactory, gustatory, visceral, and other sensory information, as well as significant input from the amygdala and other limbic regions and the rest of the prefrontal cortex. As such, it integrates visceral-sensory information with emotional affect.

Like the ventromedial region, the orbitofrontal region has a role in making appropriate social responses, especially in situations involving fear and aggression. For example, a patient who had damage to his right orbitofrontal cortex showed an impaired ability to recognize angry and disgusted faces or to recognize negative emotional reactions in others. His apparent inability to generate these expectations led to inappropriate social behaviors. The findings in this patient are consistent with results of other studies suggesting that the right orbitofrontal cortex is involved with negative emotions, and the left orbitofrontal cortex, with positive stimuli and positive social emotions. This left-positive, right-negative generalization may apply to many areas of the prefrontal cortex, although many counterexamples show it is a significant overgeneralization.

The orbitofrontal cortex is involved in choosing a response to a stimulus based on previous associations with the emotional pleasantness or unpleasantness of the consequences of the stimulus. Such functioning takes internal motivation into account and allows for situational flexibility that goes beyond simple habit. In making such choices, this part of the cortex is especially responsive to taste and flavor because it contains the secondary and tertiary taste and olfactory areas. An interesting ability this input provides is that it allows an animal to choose to avoid a particular food that it has just eaten to satiation, but still eat other food, based on the activity of neurons in this region.

In patients with damage to this area, decision-making ability is impaired. The orbitofrontal cortex also monitors the results of an action and generates signals when there is a mismatch between expectation and outcome. The loss of such information after frontal lobe damage may be part of the reason why such patients behave in socially inappropriate ways; they have no way of becoming aware of the mismatch between their intentions and the outcomes of their actions.

Obsessive-Compulsive Disorder

A major projection of outputs of the orbitofrontal cortex is to the striatal region of the basal ganglia, especially the caudate and putamen, and then to the substantia nigra. Via this pathway orbitofrontal activity can trigger and influence patterns of motor behavior based on choices such as whether or not to respond to a stimulus. Knowledge of the existence of this pathway and of its behavioral implications is the basis of new theories on the cause of OCD. Neuroimaging studies of individuals with OCD show the orbitofrontal cortex, basal ganglia, and substantia nigra to be constantly hyperactive.

OCD has two separable components, obsession and compulsion, that normally exist together. An *obsession* is a persistent idea, usually associated with a fear or doubt, that intrudes on normal cognitive activities. A person may doubt that the stove was turned off or the garage door was closed, or that a baby in the next room is still breathing, despite constant checking. The sufferer's attempts to relieve the anxiety caused by obsession lead to the compulsive action. *Compulsion* is an irrational and inordinate repetition of a behavior that interferes with normal activities of daily living. For example, compulsive fear of germs may lead to obsessive hand washing to the point of rubbing the skin raw. Fear that the front door is not locked may lead to returning to it so many times that getting far from the house is almost impossible. Interestingly, such persons may have a cognitive understanding of their problem but that does not seem to alleviate it.

Repeating a behavior over and over sounds exactly like an orbitofrontal cortex running out of control and signaling for the same action to be constantly repeated. Simultaneously, the monitoring of actions and consequences usually carried out in this area seems to be lost, possibly because of a lack of inhibitory circuits that normally turn orbitofrontal-striatal networks down and keep them in balance. Without appropriate inhibition and monitoring, an action may cause an output, which causes a response that returns a signal, which is misinterpreted and causes more response, leading to a runaway vicious cycle. This rudimentary hypothesis does not account for the known involvement of other prefrontal and subcortical regions, but at least it provides a start in understanding OCD.

INSULAR GYRUS

One other limbic area is interesting to mention. A small region called the *insular gyrus* is buried dorsal to the anterior part of the parahippocampal gyrus. It appears to integrate information from a large number of areas including visceral sensory and somatosensory cortex, amygdala, olfactory cortex, taste areas, and much of the temporal lobe. Some of its output controls cardiovascular responses to emotional stress. These effects are stronger in highly emotional people than in those with a calmer personality, a finding that has led to the suggestion that hyperactivity in the insular gyrus may be related to heart attacks.

Interlude—Acupuncture and the Limbic System

The Chinese practice of acupuncture as a healing technique stretches back over 2500 years. Its acceptance by "Western medicine" has been hindered by the lack of any "standard" physiologic explanation of its effects. The availability of brain imaging studies is now providing new information that can help validate acupuncture.

In one study, normal American subjects were scanned by MRI while the point LI4 on the hand, known as *hegu*, was treated with acupuncture needles by experienced practitioners. Pricking the same point was one of the controls used to determine brain areas specifically influenced by the treatments. Point LI4 was chosen because it is traditionally used to alleviate stress, agitation, and depression and also to achieve general analgesia.

The part of the somatosensory cortex that received input from the area stimulated was active, as would be expected from standard somatotopic maps. Simultaneously, a variety of limbic regions showed deactivation, including the amygdala, parahippocampal gyrus, anterior cingulate gyrus, hippocampus, and some brainstem nuclei. Deactivation of these areas is consistent with calming influences and a decrease in negative emotions and feelings.

Interestingly, the study exhibited a unique internal control, as follows. When acupuncture is effective, the subject experiences a condition known as *deqi*. *Deqi* involves the physical sensation of numbness, tingling, and a dull ache in and around the point of needle insertion. Eleven of the 13 subjects in the study experienced *deqi* and showed limbic system deactivation. For 2 subjects the needles did not elicit *deqi* but instead only resulted in local pain. Neither of these 2 subjects showed the deactivation of limbic structures observed in the other subjects.

It is not known exactly how the acupuncture stimulus in the hand is relayed to the limbic system. Nonetheless, the basic finding is clear and compelling, whatever the ultimate explanation.

THINKING

REVIEW

Lecture 6 began with definitions of emotions and feelings. Emotions are innate, automatic reactions that have both an autonomic, somatic component much like a motor pattern, and a conscious awareness. The fact that a small number of emotions have genetically determined expressions that accompany their conscious recognition implies they were selected for during human evolution as a basic mode of interpersonal communication. A feeling is a complex mix of emotions and thoughts about those emotions.

The brain regions responsible for emotions are among the evolutionarily oldest parts of the brain, including regions of the prefrontal cortex, cingulate gyrus, hippocampus, and hypothalamus (which are sometimes grouped together under the name *limbic cortex*). The automatic outputs of these regions comprise the parasympathetic and sympathetic divisions of the autonomic nervous system. The latter uses noradrenalin to activate the "fight or flight" reaction, while the former is more concerned with "resting and digesting."

The digestive system ("gut") contains an extensive enteric nervous system (also automatic in nature) that controls all of the muscles involved with digestion. This system can operate on its own, and also communicates with the autonomic subsystems and the cortex. It is a key source of the feedback of sensations that we consciously identify as emotional responses. The hypothalamus is the brain's major controller of the body's autonomic and endocrine activity.

The amygdala is a bilateral region of anterior temporal cortex that is predominantly involved with processing the highly negative or positive aspects of emotions, and forming memories associated with them. Olfactory cortex is also extensively interconnected with emotion centers in the cortex, giving rise to the strong emotional effects of odors. Areas of frontal cortex and cingulate gyrus are important for focusing attention on individual feelings and emotions, for emotional memory, and for integrating all of these components into appropriate social behaviors.

If you *perceive* these words, give them your undivided *attention*, and have an *intention* to keep reading, then you are enacting the topic of this lecture. At this moment a great variety of stimuli are bombarding you. These words are embedded in all sorts of other visual stimuli, perhaps including a housefly that almost caught your attention while it was flying in the periphery of your visual field. Noises from machines near the place where you are reading wax and wane, and perhaps also around you are the sounds of faint words or chirps of living things. Odors, mostly familiar but sometimes novel, are always in the air. The chair you sit in presses on your body, and clothes constantly rub against your skin. From instant to instant this plethora

of stimuli is changing, sometimes smoothly, occasionally abruptly. Amidst this chaotic swirl of stimuli you manage to keep reading. Yet, should something novel—an event that is dangerous or noteworthy or interesting—occur somewhere other than on this page, you will almost instantly shift your attention to it. If the faintest whisper of the sound of your name reaches your ears, you will look up, practically startled as much as if a firecracker just went off next to your ear. If that fly comes a bit forward in your visual field, your eyes and perhaps your head will flick in its direction, causing you to momentarily lose your place on this page.

How is all of this behavior organized by the brain? Stimuli are registered by the sense organs, but how does any one of them rise through the welter of noise and through the hierarchy of brain centers to actually become a conscious perception? Must a particular stimulus reach your consciousness to have an effect on you? How many things can simultaneously be objects of your attention, and how do you choose what to attend to out of all the possible candidates? How do your desires, motivations, and interests become intentions that guide your actions? These questions are the subject of the final three lectures. This one could be subtitled "Perception, Attention, and Intention," and continues the integration of the individual functions discussed in earlier lectures. It examines the ways the "highest" centers of your brain, the *association cortex* regions, interact with each other and with sensory and motor regions to let you be the instant-to-instant central actor in the drama described above.

ASSOCIATION CORTEX

The term *association cortex* can be used to refer to any part of the cortex that is not a primary or secondary sensory or motor area. It can be defined further as a part of the cortex that does not receive input from the primary sensory or motor nuclei of the thalamus but that receives input only from the pulvinar, lateral posterior, and medial dorsal nuclei. For example, based on this broad definition, the frontal association cortex would include the supplementary motor area, frontal eye fields, as well as the regions described in the last lecture as prefrontal. However, many workers in the field reserve the name *association cortex* for the "higher-function" regions of cortex that are heavily polysensory in terms of their inputs, such as the prefrontal cortex. Thus, the regions shaded in this figure should be understood as rough approximations of regions of association cortex.

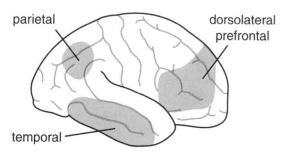

We have already met the major parts of the brain commonly labeled association cortex: ventral temporal cortex, lateral parietal cortex, and prefrontal cortex. We examined the temporal cortical regions in Lecture 3 (Sensing) as part of the "What" information stream of the visual system, discussing individual regions such as the face recognition area that malfunctions in prosopagnosics. In Lecture 5 (Communicating), we learned that defects in the temporal cortex due to localized strokes are the basis of anomias for classes of objects. In this lecture we emphasize how these parts of the temporal cortex help make sense of the visual scene and communicate with the frontal cortex to contribute to directing attention to one thing or another.

Lecture 3 presented the parietal association cortex as a component of the "where" stream of visual information. It is also a target of somatic and auditory inputs that encode the location of things in the spatial realm. This convergence of sensory inputs is an example of the basis of the word *association* in the name "association cortex." That is, in parietal association cortex, multiple sensory stimuli and their components are *associated* with each other in a process that builds an integrated concept of the location of events in space, as well as a sense of "me." In the discussion of spatial hemineglect, we saw how this process can go awry. Now, we examine how this region interacts with other brain regions in the process of paying attention to a particular thing.

Prefrontal cortex is the pivot point in the processes this lecture deals with. First, we further examine the role of the anterior cingulate cortex in directing attention. Then we emphasize the dorsolateral prefrontal cortex as the "executive" of the brain, communicating with the anterior cingulate cortex, prefrontal centers that deal with emotions, and the parietal and temporal association cortices. These interactions allow the brain to focus on and choose among alternatives, and to initiate responses.

Interlude—*A New Phrenology?*

Franz Gall (1758–1828) was a neuroanatomist who believed he could localize brain function by examining the external bulges and contours of the skull, a system he called *cranioscopy*. He attributed functions to specific regions based on his study of patients with head injuries. Gall's was a remarkably serious attempt to relate mind to brain at a time when brain function was still poorly understood. However, his idea caught the popular fancy in the early nineteenth century, was renamed "phrenology" (*phrenos* means "mind"; *logos*, "study") by its proponents, and was extended in fanciful ways. Diagrams like this one located functions such as love, cautiousness, self-esteem, and other human proclivities in early attempts at localizing brain functions.

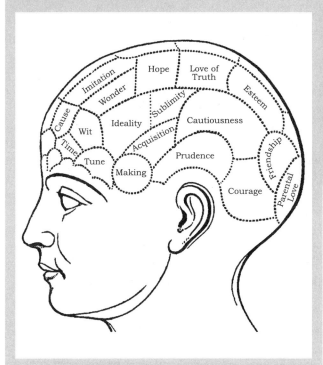

Today we view phrenology as a pseudo-science and mock its efforts. However, the attempt to localize brain functions is still a serious pursuit, moving from the domain of bony bulges to fMRI and PET scans. Indeed, much of this book discusses localization of functions.

Gall's work was a type of reductionism. He tried to *reduce* the complexity of human behavior to the functioning of individual regions of the "machine" inside the skull. This analogy is understandable, because in the age of the industrial revolution likening the brain to machinery was an obvious extension of the knowledge of the times. Now, I am concerned that we sometimes pursue "imaging reductionism," a new phrenology, either intentionally or inadvertently, depending on one's philosophical point of view.

Reductionism is especially tempting in these early days of fMRI and PET studies because only the small percentage of brain regions that are undergoing the most intense activity (or inactivity) can be discerned by these techniques. This insensitivity means that a study looking for which area is activated during function "X" often yields a localized answer. Yet, if we should learn anything from the phenomenon of parallel processing that has been discussed over and over in the previous lectures, it is that even simple functions, such as recognizing an image, involve broad regions of the cortex that are activated simultaneously. Parallel activity is true even more so for the higher functions we are dealing with in these last few lectures. In a phrase, I urge you to avoid "fMRI phrenology." Clearly, certain regions are specialized for particular functions, but the final qualities of our humanness assuredly arise from their complex, still poorly understood, parallel and interactive functioning.

EXECUTIVE FUNCTIONS

An executive in a corporation is someone who *manages*. The executive compares past experience with current inputs to make important decisions in new situations and then ensures their implementation. During your moment-to-moment activity in the world, similar functions are necessary aspects of brain activity. The executive functions of the brain are typically voluntary actions that require *thought* to solve problems and attain goals (thus the title of this lecture).

Similar to the levels of a corporation, there is a hierarchy of cortical regions, starting with primary sensory areas, moving to secondary areas, and ultimately reaching the association areas. Within those regions there is specialization, with the dorsolateral prefrontal cortex seeming to play the highest role of "executive of the cortex." We must be careful, however, not to carry the analogy too far. The brain's executive functions may depend on dorsolateral prefrontal regions, but while necessary, these regions are not sufficient. There is no little person sitting in the middle of the prefrontal cortex taking everything in and spewing out executive orders. Rather, we will see that all the association areas interact and work in parallel to achieve the brain's executive functions.

What exactly are these functions? Let us start with an example. Something unusual is happening "out there," perhaps important to your survival. You must decide which part of the sensory scene should be attended to, what response should be chosen, and what motor plan should be activated to carry it out. In doing this analysis you add the weight of past experience as well as your desires and expectations for the future.

Breaking the scenario down into even smaller subcomponents is needed in order to match tasks with brain regions. But, we do not yet know the basic properties of decision making in the same way that we can be sure of the existence of the properties of size, shape, color, brightness, and movement that make up a visual stimulus. Thus, current research dealing with the brain's executive functions depends on theories of how the brain's executive might act. These theories are postulated by cognitive scientists based on the results of psychologically oriented experiments. Note again, as in the past few lectures, how the basis of our understanding is moving further and further from easily measured sensory properties toward speculative concepts.

- Vigilance
- Selective attention
- Shift of attention
- Dealing with novelty
- Overcoming habit
- Judgment
- Planning
- Creativity
- Comparison with memory
- Holding and organizing ongoing events in working memory
- Choosing among alternative actions
- Initiating actions and sequences
- Inhibiting unwanted actions
- Regulating ongoing action
- Flexibility
- Maintenance of sense of "self as initiator"
- Monitoring outcomes
- Error correction

This table lists some of the skills and behaviors that are proposed to comprise the brain's executive functions. Listing such functions is the precursor to

searching for them. The search is done using psychological tests to see if the functions can be separated, by recording from neurons in animals, and by carrying out human neuroimaging studies to search for localization of activity during complex behaviors.

An important distinction needs to be made at the outset between *automatic* complex behaviors and *executive* complex behaviors. Ballet dancing is a complex behavior, so is driving a car, catching a ball, or playing a musical instrument. Yet, once learned, these acts require little conscious thought. Indeed, such thought can interfere with long-practiced and skilled behaviors; try thinking in detail about what you are doing the next time you tie your shoes! Executive behaviors are usually involved when a changing or novel situation requires you to recognize and select among a range of possible responses.

Change or novelty is important in triggering executive functions. Neuroimaging studies show that when such behaviors become automatic habits due to repeated occurrence, activity in the prefrontal cortex ceases to be involved. Another important difference between executive functions and complex nonexecutive ones is that the latter are not usually accessible to consciousness. Executive functions are usually voluntary and have aspects that reach consciousness, rather than simply being reflexive or automatic actions.

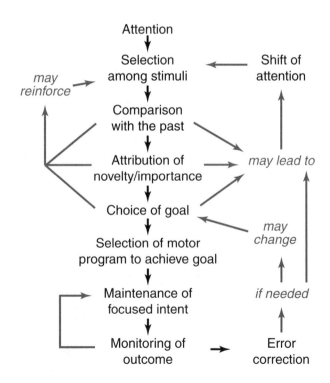

The processes in the table can be grouped into broader classes as depicted in the diagram. Those near the top of the table and the diagram involve *attention*, including selecting what should be attended to. Those in the middle involve *comparing* what is happening to the contents of memory, *choosing a goal*, and *holding it in immediate memory*. Those at the bottom of the list *inhibit interruptions*, *monitor* ongoing results, and carry out needed *error correction*. Of course, this is really a network with ongoing feedback between these activities, shown in blue in the diagram.

ATTENTION

The role of the anterior cingulate gyrus in directing emotional attention was introduced in the last lecture. It is also a key player in the generation of attention and vigilance in the executive control system. The anterior cingulate region coordinates attentional processes that arise in prefrontal, parietal, and temporal association areas during novel or difficult tasks. For example, when a person is asked to name the color and shape of a stimulus, areas of temporal association cortex involved in visual processing of color and form are activated. This activity is expected because this is the region of the "what" stream of visual information. However, if the subject is briefly shown three objects as in the next figure, first in trial 1 and then immediately after in trial 2, and must report the shape of the object that changed color, the task requires attention to multiple factors. Reflecting increased attentional needs, the dorsal part of the anterior cingulate cortex then is activated.

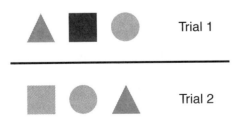

By now it should not surprise you to learn that during the classic Stroop test, when the word for a color and the color of the word do not match, the dorsal anterior cingulate area becomes active. This parallels the activation of the ventral anterior cingulate gyrus during emotional tasks such as the "emotional word" Stroop experiment discussed in the last lecture.

Parietal association areas are activated when a task requires sequential steps, especially ones involving movement. Again, when the task becomes more demanding or novel, simultaneous activation occurs in the dorsal anterior cingulate gyrus. Numerous experiments suggest that when stimuli are conflicting, cingulate neurons inhibit activity in the temporal or parietal neurons that respond to the stimuli to be disregarded.

DORSOLATERAL PREFRONTAL CORTEX

The anterior cingulate is not the only prefrontal area involved in attention; dorsal prefrontal regions also play a role. One interesting experiment that demonstrates this involves the phenomenon of binocular rivalry. To generate such rivalry, entirely different stimuli are shown in the left and right visual fields. They are adjusted in intensity so that the subject normally reports seeing only one of them, with periods when the other is briefly seen, although both activate the primary visual cortex. The moment of change from seeing one picture to the other is a moment when attention switches. Subjects reported such moments of switching, which were then correlated with the associated brain activity measured with fMRI. Anterior cingulate and dorsal prefrontal areas were activated when the switch occurred.

Other experiments involving switch of attention require subjects to covertly change their visual attention from an object in the center of their visual field to one in the periphery but without any eye movement. In such cases both dorsal prefrontal and cingulate areas are active. Interestingly, neurons in the frontal eye fields (near the back of the frontal cortex) became active, as if the eyes intended to move but did not. Taken together, a large number of studies suggest that the medial regions of dorsal prefrontal cortex are involved in monitoring general activity, while the lateral regions are more stimulus-specific in what they attend to.

When the need to choose among alternatives involves deciding among positive and negative outcomes, the anterior cingulate and dorsolateral prefrontal cortical regions interact significantly with the emotional decision areas of the prefrontal cortex, such as the orbitofrontal, as discussed in the last lecture. The principle this emphasizes is that deciding among goals is a complex procedure that involves weighing numerous factors in a process which typically requires the parallel activity of multiple networks of connections throughout the prefrontal cortex and in other association areas. No one region alone is the "decision maker."

Interlude—*Attention Deficit and Hyperactivity Disorder*

Attention deficit and hyperactivity disorder (ADHD) is a controversial condition often diagnosed as the cause of learning difficulties in young school-age children who seem unable to maintain attention on a task. Often, neuroactive drugs such as Ritalin are prescribed to quiet these hyperactive children down. However, this trend has been criticized as simply trying to make normally active young boys —who predominate in ADHD diagnosis statistics— more tractable. Thus, it would be useful to have objective neurologic tests for ADHD.

One promising group of studies involves neuroimaging. MRI and fMRI studies of children clearly diagnosed as having ADHD show lower levels of activity in the prefrontal areas involved in attention compared to those in the normal controls. Further, a prefrontal-striatum circuit involved in motor control is also affected. Specifically, there is decreased activity in regions of the basal ganglia that are normally active during situations requiring control of motor tasks.

WORKING MEMORY

Memory is a complex subject presented at length in the next lecture. Here, we need to concentrate on one aspect, *working memory*. This kind of memory is temporary and is used to keep in mind the details and procedures involved in the immediate action that is being stimulated by the attentional systems. Unlike permanent memory, which has an enormous, long-lasting storage capacity, working memory is very small, with constantly changing content.

Working memory has multiple components. Two obvious ones are the memory traces themselves

and the executive functions that manipulate these bits of memory. Further subdivisions are contained in an influential theory proposed in the 1980s by Allan Badderly. He suggested that there are separate regions in working memory to store verbal information and visual-spatial information. Further, the verbal compartment may have two subcomponents, linked in what he called the *phonological loop*; one contains the language content, and the other is a subvocalization process that constantly refreshes it. A similar rehearsal process for nonverbal working memory, called the *scratch-pad*, is also postulated. Another distinction applied to working memory is that some memories are of new, incoming information, while others are current activation of prior information that is stored in long-term memory.

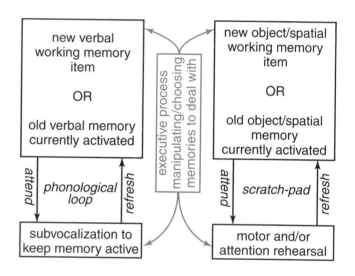

All of these ideas are represented in this diagram. Each box or process is intended to depict a different network of activity, although there is probably much overlap. Whether or not they turn out to be correct in light of further experimentation, these ideas provide a nice framework for our discussion as we look at the evidence for them and for their possible cortical localization.

LOCALIZATION OF WORKING MEMORY

The attempt to understand working memory is a very active area of research that has moved from the primary use of psychological experimentation to the use of neuroimaging to "look" at locations in the brain

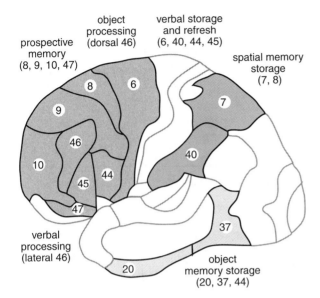

prospective memory (8, 9, 10, 47)

object processing (dorsal 46)

verbal storage and refresh (6, 40, 44, 45)

spatial memory storage (7, 8)

verbal processing (lateral 46)

object memory storage (20, 37, 44)

whose activity correlates with particular working memory tasks. The figure reproduces the map of Brodmann's areas (BA) from Appendix I. It and the following discussion are a simplified presentation intended to highlight principles related to working memory, and are not intended to be a comprehensive presentation of all that is known.

The first point to be made is that all three association areas, not just prefrontal ones, participate in aspects of working memory. For example, when the spatial location of an object is being remembered, both the parietal association area (BA 7) and the prefrontal area (BA 8) are active. When an object is being remembered, temporal visual association areas (BA 20 and 37) as well as Broca's area (BA 44) are activated. Verbal storage involves Broca's area (BA 44 and 45), as well as parietal regions (BA 40) that include Wernicke's area.

The fact that Broca's area is active in many working memory activities reinforces a point made in Lecture 4. Namely, Broca's area is not simply the language output center of the cortex. In fact, its activation in nonverbal situations reflects its evolutionary history and is the basis of its role in the later adaptation that is language. One demonstration of the multiple functionality of Broca's area is shown by the following experiment. A subject had to remember a verbal stimulus and then act on it many seconds later when a prompt was presented. The interim period of remembering prior to the prompt was compared with a control stimulus for which there was no need to make any future response. Thus, subtracting the control from the response task is

an attempt to identify the cortical regions that constitute the rehearsal portion of the phonological loop. The resulting maps showed activation of Broca's area (BA 44 and 45) and parts of the premotor cortex (BA 6) involved in speech. This activation is understood as follows. Keeping a verbal stimulus in mind involves subvocalizing it over and over, a kind of internal, silent rehearsal. This rehearsal turns out to use parts of the same network normally active when speech is actually externalized by being spoken. In retrospect this finding is not surprising, but it was not predicted when Broca's area was considered responsible simply for speech output.

BA 46 is a key region of dorsolateral prefrontal cortex and is a major component of the working memory system. Neuroimaging experiments show that it is not a site for storage of memories. Rather, it manages the executive processes that choose and maintain attention to the items from memory that are of immediate use. Its level of activation increases for tasks that require complex decision making. Further, it is subdivided such that verbal tasks are carried out in lateral and ventral portions of BA 46, while spatial tasks are carried out in its dorsal subdivision. Moreover, there may be left-right specialization as well. Some experiments suggest that BA 46 in the right hemisphere may be preferentially activated by nonverbal stimuli, while BA 46 in the left hemisphere is more sensitive to verbal stimuli. This result is consistent with the predominance of the left hemisphere in language, as discussed in Lecture 5.

The interaction of BA 46, the parietal cortex (BA 7), temporal cortex (BA 20 and 37), and anterior cingulate cortex may form a network equivalent to the object scratch-pad. This is the equivalent for objects of the phonological loop, in that it keeps refreshing a specific nonverbal object of attention. For example, the memory of an object's spatial position is maintained in the parietal cortex. The choice of attending to that remembered position over other distracting stimuli is carried out by dorsal BA 46, which inhibits the memories of objects at other positions. The anterior cingulate keeps triggering this process over and over as a way of refreshing the particular memory while it is being used.

The most frontal parts of the prefrontal cortex (BA 8, 9, 10, and 47) have been implicated in keeping in working memory the nature of a task that must be performed in the future, while disregarding distracting stimuli. This is certainly not all this large expanse of cortex does. Especially BA 10 and 47 are among the least understood part of the brain. This lack of knowledge is probably because these regions are part of networks that underlie subtle mental characteristics that are not easily described, let alone readily isolated by neuroimaging.

ERROR CORRECTION

A major component of prefrontal executive function is the temporal coordination of responses. One important part of this process is the need to monitor the results of an action in order to correct any errors. For example, suppose you intend to pick up a glass of water and start to move your arm. However, its trajectory needs to be adjusted because your body unexpectedly shifts position due to the movement.

The executive system is especially involved in tasks that require the integration of more than one sense. An example might be turning your head to look in the direction of a sudden sound and moving your eyes to see the source of the noise; vision, hearing, and motor control of muscles all need to interact appropriately. The areas of association cortex that participate in such error correction vary as a function of the task.

Error correction was studied in an experiment that used a test often employed to assess the results of injury to the prefrontal cortex. It involves a hand movement task that is difficult to perform correctly after certain kinds of prefrontal damage. The subject must repetitively close and open each hand simultaneously. However, the movements are done out of phase, so that one hand is opening while the other is closing. Finally, the motion happens while the subject looks at only one hand (e.g., the left hand).

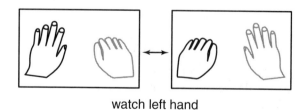

watch left hand

Normal subjects were studied during a clever manipulation of this repetitive task, as depicted in this

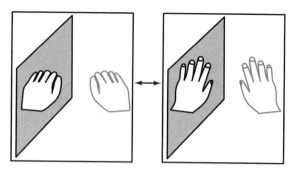

watch left side but see right hand in mirror

figure. A mirror was positioned so that while looking in the direction of the left hand, the subjects saw the mirror image of the right hand. Thus, although the subjects knew their intent was to open (or close) their left hand, they received somatic feedback that the act occurred and simultaneously received visual feedback that was entirely opposite and inconsistent. Clearly, the error correction circuits of the executive system would be highly active in monitoring this complex task.

Using PET neuroimaging and appropriate controls, researchers determined that the right dorsolateral prefrontal cortex (in the dorsal-most area overlapping the BA 9/46 border) was highly activated by the error task. Interestingly, the right side was always activated independent of whether the left or right hand was attended to. In a slightly different situation the intentional aspect of the task was removed by moving the hands passively with a motorized bar but still using the mirror to produce confounding sensations and visual perception. In this case the more ventral portion of BA 46 was most active. This finding suggests that there are subnetworks within the dorsolateral prefrontal executive area sensitive to intent mismatch versus perception mismatch.

The anterior cingulate region and the parietal and temporal association areas are also involved in error monitoring. For example, in the experiment described above, when the test condition was a simple comparison of moving both hands in phase (both opening or closing at the same time) versus out of phase, the latter more difficult monitoring task brought the parietal association area to levels of increased activity.

The role of the anterior cingulate presents an interesting variation on the error-monitoring theme, as shown by a study comparing normal subjects with patients who suffered damage to their prefrontal cortex (but not damage to any part of the cingulate gyrus).

Two tasks were used. One was simple with little need for error correction. The other was complex and required high error correction. In normal subjects the complex task generated significant activity in anterior cingulate regions and the simple one did not. In patients with prefrontal damage both tasks generated the same amount of anterior cingulate activity. Further, the amount of activity in the patients matched that of the normal subjects during the complex task. These results suggest that prefrontal areas and anterior cingulate areas are part of an error-monitoring and error correction network. The cingulate *monitors* task activity at all times, as shown by the result in the patients with prefrontal damage. The prefrontal cortex seems to be a region where a decision is made based on the cingulate's information and where corrective action is generated. When no correction is needed, the prefrontal region actually inhibits the monitoring that occurs in the cingulate, possibly because the ongoing task needs less attention than other things that might occur.

SCHIZOPHRENIA

Schizophrenia is a complex and still baffling mental disorder. It typically starts in early adult years and has a large constellation of symptoms. However, not all types of symptoms occur in all patients. A source of the puzzlement presented by schizophrenia is that a significant fraction of patients improve spontaneously, another group benefits from pharmacologic treatment, and still another group of patients does not seem to benefit from treatment and shows continuous deterioration of their mental state over a period of years. However, no reliable tests can predict which group a new patient will eventually be in. It is not even clear whether schizophrenia is a single condition or a collection of closely related ones. Understanding its basis and developing treatments are important both for the well-being of its sufferers and because of the high health-care costs of institutionalizing people with its most severe manifestations.

For approximately the first half of the twentieth century our approaches to understanding schizophrenia were primarily psychiatric. Inner impulses and distorted emotional understanding were implicated as culprits. Disruption of the normal development of these functions was postulated to be the result of inappropriate social settings and upbringing. Put another way, along the often-debated nature-versus-nurture continuum, schizophrenia was placed at the *nurture* end of the scale. With the advent of psychoactive pharmaceuticals in midcentury, some patients were treated successfully, suggesting that problems in basic brain circuitry might be at the center of the disorder. Still, the cause of "bad brain circuits" was in doubt—was it genetic-based or nurture-based?

Now, our growing understanding of the role of the prefrontal cortex in generating appropriate or inappropriate behavior is leading to new approaches to the disease. Even the way we name and understand the symptoms is changing. Hearing voices is no longer just a hallucination but instead is a breakdown in sensory processing. Other symptoms are being recast in cognitive terms and are seen as failures of executive function. It seems that the pendulum is now swinging toward the *nature* end of the nature-nurture scale to a version of "brain circuit reductionism" rather than the old "psychiatric reductionism." Eventual explanations, if we ever reach them, will probably fall somewhere in between.

ROLE OF ASSOCIATION AREAS

Some of the more interesting hints about the causes of schizophrenia can be understood in terms of the topics discussed in this lecture. In a group of remarkable studies, fMRI was used to examine the brains of people "hearing voices" in their head when no external speech was occurring. Normal subjects who imagined hearing a voice other than their own were compared to schizophrenics who were scanned at the moment they reported hearing a voice. The surprising finding is that both groups showed activation of the areas of auditory sensory cortex normally responsive to speech. However, there was a crucial difference between the normal subjects and the patients. In the normal subjects a region of the temporal association cortex that is part of the feedback monitoring network for speech was active when the inner voice was imagined. This region was not significantly active in the schizophrenics while they were hearing a voice.

We can understand these results as follows. The normal individual has an intent to generate the imagined voice. The intent activates the attentional circuits in the temporal cortex that are part of the error-monitoring circuit. So, the individual expects that a voice—his or her own—is about to be heard. When the activity in the primary auditory cortex happens, the person has all the information needed to interpret the situation. The monitoring regions of the temporal association cortex recognize first that the "sound" is not exactly like a real sound, and second that its source is the intent generated by prefrontal areas. No mistake is made in thinking that some alien voice is speaking.

In the case of the schizophrenic, the circuitry that monitors speech in the temporal cortex fails to be activated. The individual hears a voice, perhaps with a strange resonance. He or she does not have the information needed to know it is internally self-generated, and thus reports, "Someone is speaking in my head" because that is the experience actually happening! What causes the inner speech in the first place? Most likely it is part of the thinking always going on in our head.

Interlude—*Imagination*

It is not obvious why the primary auditory cortex should be activated when a person is hearing a nonexistent sound. Why should an imagined sound use the same sensory circuitry that is used for hearing real sounds? In fact, the same turns out to be true for vision. When normal subjects imagine seeing a picture in their head—in the mind's eye, so to speak—the primary visual cortex and especially the extrastriate regions starting with V2 become active. Even imagined tastes and smells activate their appropriate primary sensory regions. Clearly, a general principle is emerging. Imagination may be triggered in the association cortices, but the experience itself uses the normal sensory circuitry that the brain has already provided. I think of this metaphorically as follows. A picture that we imagine is like a photographic slide that is stored somewhere in our memory. When we choose to view it, what is more obvious than using the built-in "slide projector" in our brain, namely, the visual-sensory cortical regions?

ANATOMY OF SCHIZOPHRENIA

Many MRI studies consistently show that there is less gray matter in the prefrontal cortex of schizophrenics than in normal control subjects, as well as a decreased size in the parts of their hippocampus that directly communicate with the prefrontal cortex. Similar decreases have been observed in thalamic and basal ganglia regions that are part of input and output action networks. Interestingly, prospective, familial studies show that the appearance of these abnormalities can precede symptoms by many years. Thus, defects of early brain development may be in part responsible for eventual symptoms.

Examinations at autopsy have shown that the ratio of excitatory to inhibitory synapses in association cortex is abnormal in schizophrenics. This changed ratio suggests that the normal balance of excitation and inhibition is disrupted. Changes in synapses that use GABA and glutamate as transmitters have also been found. Clearly, schizophrenia has a basis in abnormal brain anatomy and physiology, especially involving defects in executive functions and inhibitory circuits.

The causes of these abnormalities are still unclear. Numerous studies show that a tendency to develop schizophrenia can be inherited, although the involvement of just a single gene is unlikely. Further, what is inherited seems to be a predisposition to develop the disease, rather than schizophrenia itself. Not all siblings who show similar abnormalities on MRI scans develop schizophrenia. Complicating the situation even further, cases appear that are not readily traced to inheritance. In the end, understanding the basis of schizophrenia will probably depend on unraveling the mystery of how brain structure, behavior, and personality are related in all humans, not just those with mental diseases.

THOUGHT AND INTELLIGENCE

Where do thoughts come from when you are sitting alone in a quiet room? What is the basis of intelligence and creativity? Very preliminary MRI and PET studies are focusing on the association cortex regions, especially the prefrontal cortex, to answer these questions. Again, it is important to warn that we are not searching for a "thought center" in the brain but rather must seek answers in networks of activity and interconnection.

It is conceptually difficult to examine the brain during spontaneous thinking. Such studies require neuroimaging experiments that look at the brain while "nothing is happening" and that then try to correlate activity patterns with thinking. But, how can such correlations be made? One experiment attempted to address this question with PET scans. Subjects had to carry out simple but distracting tasks that varied in their levels of distraction. Subjects were asked to report, on a scale of low to high, how many spontaneous independent thoughts occurred during the distracting tasks. As expected, more such thoughts were reported during sessions of low versus high distraction. Then, regions of brain activation were correlated with reported amount of spontaneous thought. In this way, the medial prefrontal region was identified as a possible source for initiating spontaneous thought. Clearly, this work is just a beginning in trying to understand "just thinking."

It is easier to examine the neural basis of active reasoning because logic tasks can be correlated with brain activity. Experimenters used PET scans to determine if deduction and induction utilize the same networks. The situations compared were listening to and actively trying to understand three sentences, trying to determine if a third sentence followed logically from two others (deduction), and trying to determine whether a third sentence was plausible given two others (induction). Using appropriate subtraction techniques, researchers found that deduction preferentially activates the left inferior frontal gyrus (BA 45 and 47), and induction selectively involved the left superior frontal gyrus (BA 8 and 9). At the least, these results show that reasoning itself is not a unitary process and that different kinds of reasoning utilize different prefrontal networks.

IQ

The neural basis for creativity and intelligence is one of the most controversial topics that arises when higher brain functions are considered. The ongoing debates have multiple components. First, how are intelligence and creativity defined? Second, even if they can be defined, how can these qualities of thought be measured? Third, are these the kinds of functions that are localized in specific parts of the brain, or do they involve multiple networks working in parallel? These debates have raged for over 100 years and it is clear that we still do not have answers. However, the direction

one takes in trying to approach these questions has a strong influence on the kinds of modern, neuroimaging-based experiments that are devised to study them.

In 1904 Charles Spearman proposed that there is a general factor of intelligence (g) that is the common basis of a wide range of cognitive tasks. That is, he suggested that cognitive skill is fundamentally a single kind of phenomenon. The factor g is basically equivalent to what is called *intelligence quotient* (IQ).

Given this sequence of pictures a, b, c

a   b   c

Which one of the following pictures logically completes the sequence?

The prevalence in our society of IQ tests, of which this picture is an example problem, indicates that many smart people (especially those who score well) believe that such a theory is correct. However, numerous competing theories have been put forward over the years, suggesting that there is not one general kind of intelligence but rather a collection of diverse skills (intelligence*s*) that are the basis of our intellectual abilities.

A recent experiment used PET scanning to test for the existence of g by determining how much of the cortex is active during spatial or verbal IQ-type tasks. After subtracting away sensory areas involved in perception as well as regions activated by appropriate control tasks, researchers found that the spatial intelligence task bilaterally activated a well-defined region of dorsolateral prefrontal cortex approximately centered over BA 46. The verbal task also activated this region but only in the left hemisphere. Further, the amount of activation correlated positively with task difficulty.

It is hardly surprising that intellect and prefrontal cortex are associated, as the experiment showed. Much research on patients with different kinds of prefrontal cortical damage has associated this region with intelligence and intellectual behavior. Also, the implication of intelligence arising in the prefrontal cortex is consistent with the known decline in the intelligence of long-term schizophrenics. What is surprising is the strong localization found in this experiment. Is it due to the choice of tasks? Was the possible confounding nature of the various executive processes that occur in BA 46 really controlled for? Could massive parallel processing have been missed because simultaneous, moderate activation of multiple neural networks is almost impossible to demonstrate with current neuroimaging techniques? Only more sensitive techniques that approach this question from multiple perspectives using sophisticated analytical methods will answer these questions.

TALENT AND EXPERTISE

Finally, let us examine a few ideas about talent and expertise, suggesting that their linkage is very complex. It has been known for a long time that a significant difference between a talented expert and a novice is that the expert knows "how to know" more so than does the novice. Further, the expert but not the novice recognizes useful patterns when presented with a problem, sort of like seeing the outlines of the forest, rather than being entrapped by details, akin to seeing the trees one by one.

Newer studies have shown that expertise is not all process, however. It can take as many as 5000 hours engaged in practice and relevant activities to become an expert. This need is obvious for motor expertise. Think of the endless hours of practice needed to become an Olympic-class ice skater. The need for practice also is true of intellectual expertise. When closely examined, the processes used by experts are found to draw upon an extensive memory of individual facts and previously learned patterns.

Of course, part of expertise is that facts are organized in interconnected groups relevant to their application. An interesting experiment demonstrates this principle. A novice and a chess master were allowed a quick glimpse of a chessboard in the middle of a game. The pieces were then removed and each person had to replace the pieces back on the board as accurately as possible. The novice was very inaccurate, but the master placed most of the pieces correctly. Next, the same pieces were placed on the board in legal but otherwise random positions. In that case the master did little better than the novice.

What is the difference between the two situations? The chess master literally carries the organized memories of thousands of games both personally played and intensively studied by replaying famous games of the past. When the master looked at the first board, groups of pieces were seen in well-known configurations so that the board could be said, perhaps, to resemble a known defense of a familiar opening. These patterns were easily recalled from memory when the time came to replace the pieces on the empty board. However, the random board offered no such cues. The entirely new random memorization task was no easier for the master than the novice. Clearly, much of what may seem to be remarkable intellect is more than anything else the result of long hours of practice.

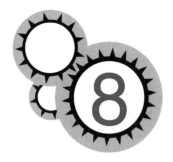

CHANGING

The previous lecture focused on the role of association areas of the cortex in thought, memory, and other "higher functions" of the brain. Temporal association areas analyze the visual stimuli, parietal association areas synthesize multiple senses into a coherent whole, and the frontal cortex originates and integrates executive functions. Executive functions, like executive roles in a corporation, are concerned with management of the thought required to attain goals, such as vigilance, attention, error correction, planning, and memory management. Working memory is used to keep track of these functions on an ongoing basis and involves large areas of—and connections between—all of the association areas.

Two main subdivisions of working memory are the verbal component: the phonological loop, and the object-in-space component: the sketch-pad. A major function of working memory is error correction, which compares the memory of what was intended with the feedback of what is happening. The prefrontal cortex is especially involved in this correction process. Schizophrenia is a mental disease in which the normal synthesis of multiple executive functions is disrupted.

Cognitive ability combines talent and expertise. Part of talent is due to innate patterns of connectivity in an individual's brain that are established during prenatal development, based on one's particular genetic makeup. After birth, experience leads to further development of talents, particularly critical reasoning skills in specific subject areas. Expertise also involves building up a large "memory bank" of individual facts that an expert uses as the objects of reasoning skills.

What happens in the brain when you learn something? Clearly there must be a physical change. Otherwise, your brain would be exactly as it was the moment before, with no trace of the new memory that resulted from learning. So, what is it that changes and how are such changes accomplished?

A fundamental premise underlies the previous paragraph. Namely, every thought, every action, and every memory are the results of physical processes and anatomic connections within the brain. If a new memory is made, the physical state of the brain must have changed to be its basis. Why? Because as far as we know, there is nothing else in your head but the physical brain that follows physical laws. Lecture 9 will have much more to say about the concepts of self and consciousness. In this lecture we examine what is known about what memory is and about how it is formed.

We need to realize at the outset that learning and memory are fundamentally intertwined concepts, even though not all memories are overtly learned. For example, we do not typically use the word *learning* to describe your memory of what you had for breakfast. Still, we will see that the processes producing a memory of events are closely related to processes involved in learning facts. Further, it will be important to understand how changes that are the basis of memory are related to those that govern the development of new connections as the brain of a baby matures after birth.

In this lecture we define memory, then examine the cellular, neuronal processes that are its substrate, and finally look at how the brain can change over the course of initial human development and throughout lifelong learning. We deal almost exclusively with long-term memory, as contrasted with short-term and working memory, which were presented in the last lecture.

STUDYING MEMORY

The study of memory has a long history in the fields of psychology and neurology. Psychologists devise tests to study what is and can be remembered. From these studies, theories of different kinds of memories have been developed. Neurologists examine patients after strokes or head trauma to see what changes occurred in the memory system. Such studies involve determining the kinds of memories that are still there, as well as the types of new memories the patient can make. To fill out our picture of how memory is studied, we need to add modern neuroimaging studies to the mix. Examination of brain activation during various learning and memory states suggests the particular brain regions involved and the patterns of connections between them.

The observations made by neurologists can become a lens through which the theories of memory put forth by experimental psychologists are examined and correlated with the results of fMRI and PET studies. Such interdisciplinary convergence is the basis of the definitions that are presented next. However, it is important to note that there are still more theories than final explanations. In fact, researchers do not even agree that the "different" kinds of memory described here are distinct from each other. Nor can they agree on hierarchies of memory function similar in kind to those put forward for motor control systems or the parallel processing systems of the visual system.

EPISODIC AND SEMANTIC MEMORY

The items in the next table are examples of *declarative memory*, which consists of the memories available to consciousness. In contrast, nondeclarative memories do not rise to the level of consciousness. For example, the learned motor skill of riding a bicycle does not involve consciously recalling muscle movements as you are riding. Two subdivisions of declarative memory are proposed. Items 1a, 2a, and 3a are examples of *episodic memory*, namely, memory of events that occurred at a particular time and place in one's own life. Besides being vignette-like episodes, they are an essential component of what we call *self*. They happened to "me" and are part of the stream of consciousness that makes me real to myself and different from

---

1a - I was in my yard last September and saw a squirrel bury a nut. A bluejay on a nearby branch swooped down immediately after the squirrel left and retrieved the nut. This was my introduction to the fact that jays steal from squirrels.

1b - Bluejays let squirrels do the work of finding nuts and then steal the nuts after they are buried.

2a - I remember a Halloween party I had in our apartment when I was 8 years old. It was the first time I ever tried bobbing for apples and I still recall how difficult it was.

2b - Bobbing for apples is hard because they float away as you try to bite them.

3a - I visited Madison, Wisconsin, to attend a meeting some years ago. I remember being surprised that the state capitol building was so close to the university campus.

3b - The capital of Wisconsin is Madison.

---

the world around me. Sometimes the ability to remember the facts embedded in such memories is inextricably tied to the recall of the entire episode.

Examples 1b, 2b, and 3b exemplify *semantic memory*, which is knowledge of concepts and facts that is not tied to any particular episodic scene, time, or place. The fact that you can rattle off a list of state capitals memorized for a test long ago without any memory of when, where, or how you memorized them is semantic memory at work.

The phonological loop and the object/spatial sketch-pad, discussed in the last lecture, are considered to be precursors of episodic and semantic memory. For example, the phonological loop recognizes phonemes, which other systems build into words with meanings. The loop and sketch-pad result in learning through experience and thus are a kind of memory.

In both episodic and semantic memory, activation occurs in places in the brain where memories about things we can explicitly declare out loud are stored. So, why are these two kinds of memories distinguished from each other? Are they basically different? The next Interlude shows that injury and disease can selectively affect episodic or semantic memory, thus providing strong support for the distinction between them.

Interlude—*The Cases of H.M. and K.C.*

A patient identified as H.M. probably has the most famous case of amnesia ever reported, because of both the rareness of his situation and the great number of studies that have been published in which he is the subject. In 1953, when he was 27, he underwent radical brain surgery in an attempt to relieve him of debilitating, recurring epileptic seizures that were not manageable in any other way. The surgery involved removing large portions of his medial temporal lobe in both hemispheres, including the front two-thirds of his left and right hippocampus. Little was known at the time about the anatomy of memory.

His normal intellect was unimpaired after recovery from the surgery. However, he displayed a remarkable defect that changed his life forever. Namely, he was unable to form new declarative memories, either episodic or semantic, a condition called *anterograde amnesia* (the opposite of *retrograde amnesia*, in which past memories are lost).

H.M. could still readily recall past memories and facts, but for him time stopped on September 1, 1953, the day of the surgery. He still had the ability to make short-term, working memories that spanned a few minutes. However, these memories never become long-term ones. For example, his doctor introduced herself each time she visited and H.M. behaved as if it were the first meeting, even after many years of visits. Perhaps more bizarre, even when he realized that something was wrong, each time that realization occurred was new to him; he could not remember that he could not remember!

In 1981, a patient named K.C. had a motorcycle accident at age 30. He suffered severe damage to the medial temporal and frontal regions of his brain that left him with a severe amnesia different from H.M.'s amnesia; namely, he became unable to remember any episode from any time in his life or to form memories of new episodes. However, his recall of facts and concepts is not impaired and he can learn new facts. He just cannot remember where or how he learned them. In simple terms, K.C. has lost episodic memory but not semantic memory. In contrast, some patients with Alzheimer's disease, which impairs memory, have relatively normal episodic memory but great trouble remembering facts, such as the uses of a specific object.

PROCEDURAL MEMORY

Walking and running

Riding a bicycle or motorcycle

Throwing a ball accurately

Playing the piano

Pavlovian conditioning

These are examples of procedural memories, which normally are not consciously perceived and typically involve motor tasks. A basis for discriminating procedural from declarative memory is that individuals with amnesia that involves their declarative system can still learn new procedural tasks, even without being aware they are doing so. Patient H.M. provides an example, but before discussing his case, we must introduce a puzzle game.

The game called "Towers of Hanoi" requires that the player move the pieces (flat disks of different

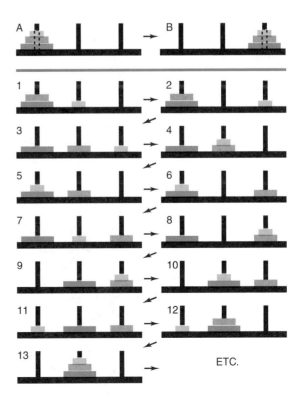

sizes with central holes) one at a time to get from the position shown in Figure A to that in Figure B. The rules are as follows: only one piece can be moved at a time; a piece can only be moved to an adjacent tower; a larger piece can never be placed on top of a smaller piece. Steps 1 through 13 show a sequence that is the beginning of a solution. If you look carefully, you will note that there is an underlying repetitive sequence of movements that accomplishes the task most efficiently. Sometimes a player comes to consciously recognize the sequence and becomes very fast at what is essentially a repetitive motor task. Other players become faster without ever consciously being able to state the sequence. Such practice effects become even more evident when four or five disks are used instead of three.

H.M. was introduced to this game and was able to hold the rules in working memory. He was given time to play. Later he was shown the puzzle again and claimed to have no memory of ever playing with it. Again he was told the rules and allowed to play. This went on for many days, with still no memory on his part from day to day that he was repeating the same game. However, over the course of time he became progressively faster at solving the puzzle. That is, even though he could not make new declarative memories about the game, as a result of practice he was able to develop procedural memory of his motor manipulations that improved his performance of the task.

The last item on the list that started this section is "Pavlovian conditioning," named after the famous Russian psychologist who first demonstrated it. Recall that he showed a dog a bowl of food and the dog would salivate in anticipation of eating. Next, a bell was rung just before the food was exposed to the animal's view. The sequence was repeated many times. Eventually, the dog would start to salivate when the bell rang, even before the food was revealed.

Stated technically, the dog was *conditioned* to *associate* the bell with the probable arrival of food. Such conditioning does not require the subject to make a conscious association between the two stimuli. Indeed, in subtle tasks a person can develop the association and never know why. It is the lack of conscious realization that places associative conditioning in the procedural memory classification. However, there is an important difference between such association and a task like riding a bicycle. Namely, the subject may be perfectly conscious of both stimuli, in a declarative sense, even though the association is built procedurally. Such

interaction of declarative and procedural memories raises questions about whether they are really totally different kinds of memory, and if they are, about how interactions may occur between them. Questions like these still await answers.

IMPLICIT MEMORY

Improvement in performance due to learning during repetition of the Towers of Hanoi puzzle exemplifies implicit memory. *Implicit memory* is most broadly defined as material that is learned without awareness that learning is occurring. Some workers in the field consider implicit memory to be synonymous with nondeclarative memory. However, given the subtleties just discussed regarding procedural memory, it is probably useful to withhold judgment. Here is an example, involving implicit memory processes, that highlights the issue. Try to complete this fragment of a crossword puzzle.

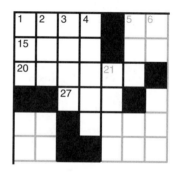

ACROSS
1. Walking aid
15. Gone wrong
20. Charge a battery
27. Simian

DOWN
1. Automobile
2. Amaze
3. Star or car
4. Run to wed

How did you generate the answers? Was every answer the result of a conscious memory search that used a clear procedure, or did some of the answers just "jump into your awareness"? Probably some of both. For those answers that simply "came to you," you have no idea what went on inside your brain to retrieve them, and memory theorists can do little better in providing an explanation. (Puzzle answers are at the bottom of page 88.)

Interlude—Who Was That Masked Man?

All of us have the experience of trying, unsuccessfully, to remember a name. For example, who was the actor most associated with playing the Lone Ranger in the early TV series? Or, what was the name of the actor who played his companion Tonto? If you know the answer, that's great. But you might not recall it, although you may have known at one time. So, you try to recall and eventually stop trying and go on to other things. Later, perhaps after a night's sleep, the answers suddenly pop into your head: Clayton Moore, Jay Silverheels! What was going on all that time between the questions and the answers? Was some neural "hard disk" churning away, testing your memory banks one item at a time? Even such a basic question about recall is beyond our current understanding. However, here is another remarkable aspect of the remembering phenomenon: Why is it that the "wrong" answer rarely pops into your head? What "filter" in the brain only allows the correct answer through? (Yes, sometimes you get the last name right but have the first name wrong. However, we all have the experience of fully recognizing that the incorrect first name "feels" wrong.)

Among the most interesting demonstrations of implicit memory are those involving the learning of "artificial grammars." First, a string of letters is prepared, such as VRNNTRG. It is developed using a predetermined, complete set of rules called an *artificial grammar*. For example, rules in such a grammar might be as follows: no letter can appear more than twice in a row; an R is always preceded by a V or a T; and so on. A subject is then instructed to memorize a group of such letter strings. After they are memorized, the subject is told that each letter sequence followed the rules of the same artificial grammar but is not told what the rules are. The subject is then shown new strings of letters and asked to judge whether they follow the grammar rules or not. Most subjects are able to correctly classify these new strings at above-chance levels, even though they cannot declaratively describe the rules of the grammar.

An interesting elaboration of this procedure involved the use of functional neuroimaging. The number 1, 2, or 3 was presented on a screen and the subject had to press the corresponding number on a keypad. Numbers were presented in long sequences. Unknown to the subject the sequences were structured by an underlying and complex artificial grammar. The subject repeated the task, and reaction time of the keypad presses was monitored. Over the course of many repetitions the latency of the subject's reaction time decreased significantly. That is, the subject was learning the grammar and correctly anticipating the next element to be presented. When little further improvement occurred, the next trial presented the number 1, 2, or 3 again but following a different set of grammar rules. The subject's reaction times suddenly increased, indicating that the prior practice no longer helped the responses to the new grammar. Of course, after testing, the subject reported being unaware of any set of rules governing the sequences or of a change in those rules. PET scans were taken simultaneously with the task. Three areas of the cortex showed a change in activity when the grammar was changed, the greatest change being found in the ventral striatum. To summarize: the subject was not conscious of patterns in the presentations; however, changes were occurring in portions of the cortex that dealt with implicit memories and those regions were extremely sensitive to differences based on comparing a new task with those memories.

PRIMING

A phenomenon known as *priming* is considered to be based in the nondeclarative memory systems. A typical test might go as follows: for each of the following three-letter prefixes, right now, you the reader should immediately say the first word that comes to mind: art-, rag-, sub-, tra-.

In a priming test, before being shown these word stems, the subject is given a very long list of words to read quickly, without making any effort to memorize them. In fact, to inhibit memorization the subject is told that the task is to try to finish reading the list as quickly as possible. Lack of memorization can be shown by the fact that when later asked if a particular word was on the list, subjects are not very accurate in their responses. However, when asked to complete the word stems, subjects respond with a word from the previously read list significantly more often than they would by chance. Such priming may even have happened for you for the stems presented above. For example, the word *subject* was used many times on the preceding pages. Did you happen to say it as your response to its stem? Priming demonstrates that there is information in memory that is difficult to access, such as the words on a list recently read. However, by priming the response, a kind of mental pointer is generated to that information and access to that memory is facilitated.

To generalize, memory about something may fail because no trace of that item or event was ever formed (as in amnesia, or for a telephone number that you remember only long enough to dial), or because even though the memory is "in there," you are unable to access it easily. A large number of experiments have demonstrated that for many things a person once knew but can no longer recall, inability to access the memory rather than degradation of the memory trace is the problem. How might such a thing be proved? By using a priming experiment, of course!

ANATOMIC LOCALIZATION OF MEMORY

A combination of fMRI and PET neuroimaging experiments, as well as localization of brain damage after strokes and injuries, allows correlations of memory processes with particular brain structures. However, making these correlations is still a crude undertaking, dependent on the model of memory that is used. For example, the next figure shows a "taxonomy" of memory that attempts to present the aspects discussed thus far in a unified scheme. Realize, however, that it is sketchy, provisional, and biased by my interpretations. (*Blue lines signify interaction; black lines, subdivisions.*)

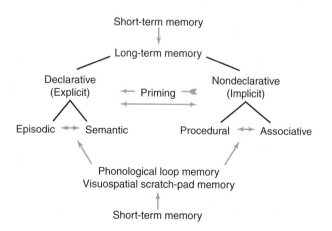

To briefly summarize, short-term memory is a stage that precedes and feeds into long-term memory. Declarative and nondeclarative memory interact, presumably unidirectionally via priming and in both directions in other memory activities. The subdivisions themselves also interact, but the details of the exact nature of such interactions are still sparse. Short-term memory also provides input to the phonological loop and the sketch-pad (discussed in the last lecture), which themselves can lead to long-term storage of the recognition factors that are a basis of their functioning. The loop and sketch-pad also provide input to declarative and nondeclarative memory. With this brief summary in hand, we can now look at the brain regions that are associated with these aspects of memory.

HIPPOCAMPUS

The hippocampus was introduced in the last lecture as an important structure in short-term, working memory. It is shown on the right side of the next figure, which is an enlargement of the region outlined by dashes on the left, made a few centimeters in from the brain's medial surface. We now need to take a more detailed look at it because it is a central player in all memory systems.

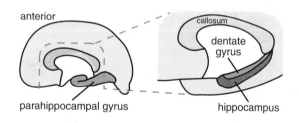

Recall that the surgery H.M. underwent removed most of his hippocampus in each hemisphere. He still retained short-term memory but could not form long-term memories. His loss, as well as the results of many other experiments, show that the hippocampus is needed for the consolidation of short-term memories into long-term memories. However, the absence of the hippocampus in H.M. shows that it is not needed for the occurrence of short-term memory itself. Further, the fact that H.M. could "learn" the Tower of Hanoi problem is one example of many findings that suggest the hippocampus is not necessary for the formation and storage of the implicit type of long-term memories.

Neither short-term nor long-term memories reside in the hippocampus; however, it is absolutely necessary for the formation of new, explicit long-term memories. Surrounding regions of the temporal cortex, including the parahippocampal and dentate gyri, have been suggested to be regions where long-term memories are stored. Other temporal areas, as well as cortical regions not in the temporal lobe, especially the association cortex, are also probable storage sites.

Some neuroimaging studies show that the hippocampus is active when explicit memories are being retrieved. Such activity seems inconsistent with the findings just described. However, closer examination shows that only recent memories are involved. That is, while memories are undergoing consolidation into long-term storage, the hippocampus is still used to access them.

Interlude—*What Hit Me?*

Teaching on a university campus, I have met more than my share of students who were involved in bicycle collisions with cars. Some were knocked unconscious but quickly recovered, with only "road rash" as a reminder of the accident. And I do mean *only*. Typically, when the victim was rendered unconscious, he or she simply did not remember what happened. In some cases memories of the time immediately prior to the accident were also missing. What's going on?

The loss of consciousness seems to interfere with the normal functioning of the hippocampus. Thus, the short-term memory of the accident was never consolidated into long-term memory. Apparently, in severe situations, memories of the most recent past that were still actively being stored are also vulnerable and get "erased."

OTHER CORTICAL AREAS

PET studies of the role of the prefrontal cortex in memory show that when complex, explicit memories are encoded, the *left* dorsolateral prefrontal cortex is activated. These experiments also show that the *right* dorsolateral prefrontal cortex is active when explicit memories are being retrieved. These findings make another general point. The memory system has three fundamental aspects: the process of initial storage (encoding), the maintenance of the memory trace over time, and access to memories that are stored. Failure of any one of these aspects is called *forgetting*. However, there are clearly different kinds of forgetting. For example, recent research using priming-type experiments showed that adults who studied a foreign language in high school but then never used it can still recall a great deal of vocabulary. However, they can only do so when the recall is primed, such as with visually presented word stems that are shown too briefly for the subject to be consciously aware of them. So, here the situation is not that the memories of the foreign vocabulary simply faded away. Rather, access to them was seriously weakened.

The left-versus-right hemisphere difference noted above is just one of many hemispheric asymmetries that are related to memory processes. For example, memory for faces, discussed earlier in Lecture 3 when prosopagnosia was described, seems to be more lateralized in the right temporal cortex. In contrast, some types of language memories are preferentially stored in the left hemisphere.

The motor memories that are the prototype of implicit memory involve numerous parts of the motor system that were discussed in Lecture 5, including the striatum in the basal ganglia, the cerebellum, and the prefrontal motor areas. Involvement of these areas in procedural memories is not surprising because such memories can readily be considered to be learned motor skills. The relationship of these areas to motor memory also explains the fact that Huntington's disease patients show a deficit in their ability to learn new motor tasks. Such inability is consistent with the pathology that appears in the basal ganglia of these patients.

CELLULAR BASIS OF MEMORY

The concept of a *memory trace* is used repeatedly in the preceding discussion as a way to refer to the specific changes in the brain that encode a new memory. What exactly does "memory trace" mean in cellular terms? When action potentials were becoming understood in the 1940s, one theory put forward was that a memory was some kind of circulating, persistent pattern of neuronal firing, constantly resonating through the cortex. However, for some patients in comas, EEG studies showed that the cortex is almost completely silent for a time. The ability of memories to persist after a coma is evidence against any simple electrical basis for memory.

At the other end of the scale from transient electrical currents, DNA is probably the stablest form of information storage in an organism. Thus, it is no surprise that changes in DNA structure were proposed as a basis of the storage of memories. This idea was strengthened by the repeated observation in experimental animals that blockade of protein synthesis keeps new memories from being formed. However, no mechanism of a memory process that changes the DNA in neurons is known. We will see, however, that the protein synthesis observation provides a vital clue.

The concept of a new memory trace means that something in the brain has physically changed. What might that be in cellular terms? Almost all current theories point to one answer: changes in synaptic strength. Remember from Lecture 1 that the postsynaptic signal at a synapse, the EPSP or IPSP, is a small graded change of a few millivolts. If somehow the size of this signal could be permanently changed, such a change could be a correlate of memory storage. How might a change occur? There are a number of possibilities that could lead to a change in synaptic strength, as described next.

1. When an action potential invades any one bouton, the probability that a synaptic vesicle will be released is usually less than 100%, typically ranging between 20% and 70%. If the density of calcium channels in the presynaptic membrane is increased, or if the calcium channels are altered in some way so as to increase their conductivity, such alterations could change the probability of vesicle release.

2. The size of the postsynaptic potential (PSP) is a function of how many vesicles are released per action potential. At many central nervous system synapses, the number is one, presumably reflecting the density of specialized release sites. Changing the density of the release sites could alter the number of vesicles released.

3. The size of the PSP depends on how many neurotransmitter molecules are released, which is a function of vesicle size. Although tightly controlled, vesicle size could be altered.

4. PSP size depends on how many postsynaptic receptors are activated by bound transmitter molecules. Thus, changing the density of postsynaptic receptors would change the size of the PSP. Similarly, altering the existing channels to change their conductivity would accomplish a change in PSP size.

5. The conductivity of the dendrite that receives a synapse could be altered. This change is most likely to happen at synapses on dendritic spines, since it is known that the morphology of the spine neck, and thus its conductivity, can be changed as a function of use.

6. Existing axonal terminal branches and dendritic trees may form new synapses. Such sprouting is a demonstrated phenomenon, although its link to learning is yet to be proved.

Presently, there is some evidence for each of these mechanisms, especially for number 4, which will be discussed next. However, it is important to stress that while extensive evidence supports the concept that synapses can change strength, there is still little compelling evidence that changes specifically occur during learning.

LONG-TERM POTENTIATION

Long-term potentiation (LTP) has been studied extensively since its discovery in the 1970s. In fact, the study of LTP may have produced more papers in the last 10 years than any other single subject (a rate of one paper per day). LTP was discovered first in the hippocampus and has since been demonstrated at excitatory synapses throughout the cortex that use the transmitter glutamate. Whatever its role in memory, LTP is clearly a mechanism used to "tune" synaptic strength and thus is important to understand. There are a number of variants of LTP. Only one is described here, and it was chosen because it has most of the properties of the phenomenon.

The next figure presents a generalized and simplified picture of the basic finding. A typical experiment usually uses a slice of brain taken from a rat. A neuronal soma and two of its dendrites are shown at the top. Three synapses on dendritic spines (*A*, *B*, and *C*) are depicted. Each receives an input from a different

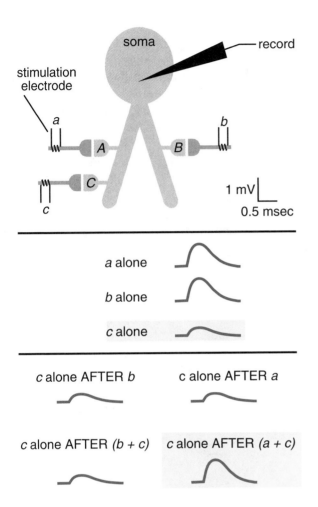

a alone

b alone

c alone

c alone AFTER b   c alone AFTER a

c alone AFTER (b + c)   c alone AFTER (a + c)

presynaptic neuron, labeled *a*, *b*, and *c*. The black stimulation electrodes represent the fact that *a*, *b*, or *c* can be electrically stimulated, either alone or in pairs. A micropipette-type electrode inside the soma is used to record the EPSPs that result from the stimulation.

The middle section shows the responses that are elicited from *A*, *B*, and *C*. Synapses *A* and *B* respond with a large EPSP, and *C* responds with a much smaller EPSP. The next part of the experiment is the control. Input *b* is stimulated repetitively at a high rate for a few seconds. After this stimulation of *b*, the response of *C* is tested and shows no change (*bottom section, upper left*). The experiment is repeated, but this time a high rate of stimuli is simultaneously applied to *b* and *c*, and then *C* is tested alone. Again, the size of the EPSP it causes shows no change (*bottom section, lower left*).

Now comes the critical test. Input *a* is stimulated repetitively at a high rate for a few seconds. After stimulation of *a*, the response of *C* is tested and shows no change (*bottom section, upper right*). Finally, a high

rate of stimuli is applied simultaneously to *a* and *c*, and then *C* is tested alone. Note that *C* now produces a large EPSP that is a substantial change from its original state, as can be seen by comparing the two responses highlighted by the light blue background. Further, if *C* is subsequently tested alone over a period of hours, its response continues to be the new, large EPSP.

What has happened? Somehow the strong stimulation of a nearby postsynaptic spine *A* at the same time as the stimulation of the weaker postsynaptic spine *C* causes an increase in the subsequent response of *C* alone. In the jargon of the trade, the simultaneous stimulation is said to *potentiate* the response of *C*. Further, this potentiation only has to occur once, after which the response of *C* remains increased for a *long term*, hence, the name of the phenomenon, *long-term potentiation*, or *LTP*. It is important to note that just intense activity of *A* does not cause LTP; the stimulation must occur simultaneously with that of *C*. Also, the control experiment shows that only activity in synapses very near to *C* can cause LTP; activity in *B*, on a different dendrite, could not.

LTP is presented in detail because it is a clear circumstance of a change in synaptic strength due to use. How *might* LTP relate to learning? An examination of a very simplified example of classic conditioning, depicted in the figure on the next page, provides a possible example. Realize it is an oversimplified, hypothetical example and that many researchers are trying to prove that something like it actually happens.

Panel (1) lays out the basic situation. Neurons *a* to *e* are shown making (presynaptic) and receiving (postsynaptic) excitatory synapses, symbolized by small circles. Synapses that are darkly filled (*dark blue or black*) are strong enough to cause the postsynaptic cell to fire an action potential. A synapse that is not filled, such as the synapse labeled *1*, does not cause an EPSP that is strong enough to generate an action potential in the postsynaptic cell.

Neuronal elements shown in light gray are meant to indicate that the cells in the figure also participate in other interactions and circuits that are not related to the functions discussed here. Their presence makes an important point. Namely, memory is probably embodied in a network of synaptic interconnections, not in specific neurons. Thus, any one neuron can participate in more than one such network.

Panel (2) shows that neurons *a* and *b* and the synapses *4*, *5*, and *6* encode a memory for some

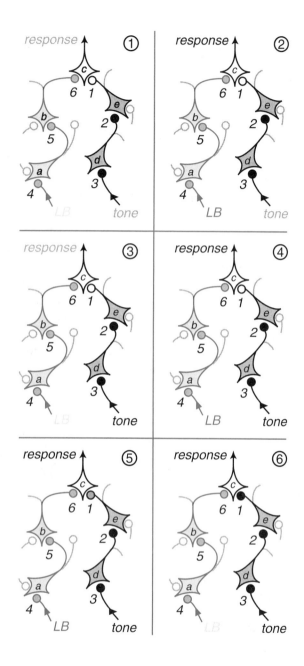

A *response* is caused in neuron *c* because synapse *6* is strong enough by itself to cause such firing. Panel (5) shows another effect of the simultaneous inputs to neuron *c* by the *LB* and *tone* pathways. Namely, synapse *1* is being strengthened by LTP, brought about by its simultaneous activation with nearby strong synapse *6*. Panel (5) shows that LTP has partially strengthened synapse *1* (*now gray instead of clear*). Further repetition of the pairing of *LB* and *tone* strengthens the LTP of this input further until, as shown in Panel (6), it becomes strong enough so that the *tone* itself is able to cause the *response*. To summarize, the *LB* pathway and the *tone* pathway have become associated by the process of LTP.

MOLECULAR BASIS OF LTP

What underlying physical change at a synapse is the basis of LTP? A number of mechanisms have been proposed, and different ones probably occur for different types of LTP. A *model* for associative LTP that incorporates many experimental results is shown in figure at

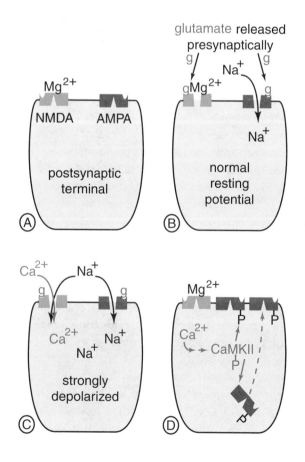

previous learned behavior, called *LB*. Thus, whenever input *LB* is activated, it causes neuron *a* to fire an action potential, activating synapse *5*, which causes neuron *b* to fire. The action potential in *b*, in turn, activates synapse *6*, which causes neuron *c* to fire, bringing about some kind of *response* in the organism. Panel (3) shows that a new stimulus, a sound *tone*, causes the firing of neurons *d* and *e*. However, synapse *1*, from *e* to the response neuron *c*, is too weak to cause an action potential in *c*.

Next, look at Panel (4), which shows the input *LB* and the input *tone* occurring at about the same time.

the bottom of the previous page. (Stress is put on the word *model* because there are still many details to be worked out.) Panel (A) shows a postsynaptic terminal that has two different types of receptors for the neurotransmitter glutamate. Their names, NMDA and AMPA, are derived from the fact that they were first identified because they selectively bind substances that mimic glutamate when applied by experimenters using pipettes. (NMDA is N-methyl-d-aspartate. AMPA is alpha-amino-3-hydroxy-5-methyl-4-isoazolepropionate.)

When glutamate is released by the presynaptic bouton, it diffuses across the synaptic cleft and binds to both types of receptors, as shown in Panel (B) (*blue g*). The AMPA receptor opens and allows sodium to enter the postsynaptic terminal, generating a small EPSP. The NMDA channel does not allow sodium to enter because it is blocked by a magnesium ion bound ionically to a specific site on its outer surface.

Panel (C) shows a different situation in which the postsynaptic dendrite is already strongly depolarized due to the action of simultaneously active, nearby synapses—the precursor condition for LTP. The strong depolarization causes the positively charged magnesium ion to unbind from the NMDA receptor. The unblocked channel now allows sodium to flow in, adding to the sodium entry through the AMPA channel. More important, the NMDA receptor has another property, different from that of the AMPA receptor. Namely, it allows calcium to flow through the channel and enter the postsynaptic dendrite. The calcium entering via the NMDA channel acts as the messenger bringing about the physical change in the dendrite that is the basis of LTP. A series of intermediate metabolic reactions, catalyzed by the calcium, lead to the phosphorylation of a molecule known as CaMKII (calmodulin kinase II). The phosphorylation makes CaMKII-P active for a long period of time, even after the calcium that entered is pumped out.

Terminology note: When a molecule such as CaMKII is phosphorylated this is indicated by appending the letter *P* to its name, making it CaMKII-P. The symbol *P* in the figure also indicates a phosphorylated molecule.

The CaMKII-P brings about two effects. First, it phosphorylates AMPA receptors already in the postsynaptic membrane. Such phosphorylated receptors allow more sodium to enter per glutamate activation than occurs with nonphosphorylated AMPA receptors, leading to an increase in the size of the EPSP. Second, via a series of steps that ultimately requires protein synthesis, CaMKII-P causes new, phosphorylated AMPA receptors to be inserted into the postsynaptic membrane. The extra receptors provide more channels that are opened per synaptic event, also leading to an increase in the size of the EPSP. Together the two changes are why the EPSP is strongly potentiated in LTP. The fact that the extra AMPA receptors and the phosphorylation persist for long periods of time is the basis of the long-term aspect of LTP. However, whether these changes are long-lasting enough to be the basis of memories that persist for years is still in question.

LTP can decay because over time there is a natural loss of the extra receptors in the postsynaptic membrane. However, the larger, potentiated EPSPs help release magnesium from its blockade of the NMDA channel during the arrival of subsequent synaptic inputs at this terminal. Thus, once potentiated, as long as the synapse continues to be activated, calcium enters and renews the potentiated state. In terms of memory, if the synapse is part of a memory trace, potentiation of the synapse is reinforced every time the memory is recalled.

SYNAPTIC PLASTICITY

The ability of neurons in the brain to make new connections and to reorganize existing ones is termed *plasticity*. The term's use is based on the meaning of plastic as being changeable or malleable. Learning and memory are forms of plasticity. However, the actual synaptic changes are difficult to observe with current techniques because the changes are distributed and subtle.

Plasticity has been observed in two other situations, both involving sensory systems. One involves looking at the early maturation of neuronal connections in neonates. The other deals with changes in sensory systems of adults after significant changes in sensory input. Current models suggest that both neonatal and adult plasticity is based on similar cellular mechanisms. However, experiments have shown that additional or different mechanisms are used in adult animals in certain situations.

DEVELOPMENT IN SENSORY SYSTEMS

The next figure depicts idealized presentations of what are now considered two classic demonstrations of synaptic plasticity during early development. Both involve manipulations of the visual environment of kittens. Kittens are particularly useful subjects for such experiments because their cortical visual system is immature when they are born and matures over the first few postnatal months.

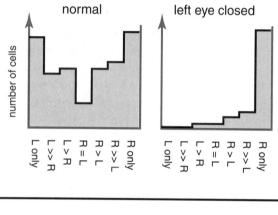

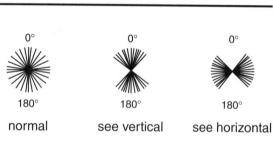

The upper-left histogram illustrates typical findings from the recording of individual neurons in V1 (BA 17), the primary visual cortex of adult cats. Many of these cells receive inputs from both eyes. The histogram shows the exact details of the pattern of these inputs. "L only" and "R only" indicate cortical neurons that receive input from only one eye. Overall, they are in the minority. All other cells receive binocular input, the middle bar showing cells in which the influence of the right and left eye inputs are equal (R = L). The other bars indicate cells with binocular input in which the input from one eye is stronger than that from the other. Note the approximately equal number of cells more strongly innervated by either of the eyes.

The histogram at the top right shows the results of the same type of recording in an animal that had the lids of its left eye sewn shut from birth. Thus, that eye never was stimulated by visual patterns, although a small amount of diffuse light penetrated the closed lids. The left lids were opened and the animal was behaviorally tested when it was adult. It was functionally blind when looking through the left eye but responded visually through the right eye. The cellular basis of the blindness is demonstrated in the histogram. Note that very few cells were responsive to left-eye stimulation. Further experiments showed that the axonal inputs to this area of the cortex that corresponded to right-eye input, from relay cells in the thalamic, lateral geniculate nucleus (LGN), increased their axonal terminal arbors by sprouting extra boutons and displacing the nonfunctional inputs that carried input from the occluded left eye.

Putting the results in plasticity terms, we can generalize as follows. The connections made by axons from the LGN onto their targets in V1 are still able to grow and change targets significantly in the neonatal animal. Boutons that carried left-eye information were relatively inactive because the animal was not allowed to see out of that eye as a kitten. Such synapses were unable to strengthen and stabilize their contact with cortical cell dendrites. The boutons driven by right-eye input were constantly trying to make as many active synapses as possible. Thus, they took over the dendritic territory that normally received left-eye input. They could do so because during the final development of connectivity, their axon terminal branches were constantly sprouting new boutons, a sign of their plasticity. Normally, inputs driven by an active left eye would also be competing in this way, and the two eyes would reach a kind of truce, represented by the equilibrium shown in the upper-left histogram. In the deprivation case, the occluded eye loses out.

The lower three polar histograms show the typical results of a different type of visual deprivation experiment. Kittens were raised in a controlled environment, continuously wearing special goggles that allowed some of them only to see vertical lines and others only to see horizontal lines. After the kittens grew up, the goggles were removed and their visual perception was behaviorally tested. Interestingly, animals raised seeing only vertical lines were totally unresponsive to stimuli that were horizontally elongated. The animals raised seeing only horizontal lines had the complementary defect; namely, they were functionally blind to vertically elongated stimuli.

Recall from Lecture 3 (Sensing) that neurons in the primary visual cortex are responsive to elongated stimuli, and that all orientations are represented in a set of adjacent cortical columns. The lower-left polar histogram depicts such a normal situation. It shows the best angle of orientation of the most effective bar stimulus for a large number of cells. The other two histograms show the results of similar recordings from animals that were only allowed to "see vertical" or to "see horizontal" when they were kittens. Note that no cortical neurons responded to orientations not seen during neonatal development. That is, an animal shown only vertical lines had no cortical neurons tuned to horizontal orientations.

You might recognize that such a change is analogous to the monocular deprivation experiment. There, inputs (via the LGN) from the deprived eye did not develop connections in the primary visual cortex. In the goggle deprivation case, the synaptic connections that are needed to organize the neuronal circuitry for neurons tuned to a particular stimulus orientation did not develop if that orientation was never seen.

To summarize, we can note that there is extensive synaptic plasticity available to the newborn visual system. It is used to generate connections that are based on what the animal actually sees. Normally, the plasticity results in a normal, stereotyped set of connections that are similar from animal to animal. However, when early stimulation is abnormally skewed or disrupted, neurons do the best they can to rewire according to what is actually seen. Further, once development is over, experiments show that recovery cannot occur, even if the visual environment is then normal.

Interlude—*Visual Deprivation in Humans*

Humans can have visual defects at birth that cause the development of abnormal circuitry in their visual cortex. However, the sensitivity of babies to such deprivation is less than that for lower vertebrates. Nonetheless, it is interesting to examine the degree to which the young human visual system can display plasticity in skewed environments. It is obviously unethical to rear newborn humans in an environment with all horizontal or all vertical stimuli. Thus, to know if the human visual system would behave similarly to that of the kitten, a "natural experiment" had to be carried out.

Researchers hypothesized that humans who grew up in an environment that was greatly deficient in vertical stimuli might show less visual acuity in the vertical than the horizontal axis. They chose to examine Canadian Inuit adults who grew up and lived in polar regions where there are no trees. Also, their environment had few constructed vertical edges, such as in rooms or buildings. Even their dwellings were either round or tent-like.

The people agreed to act as subjects and their visual optics were adjusted with lenses to correct for any optical astigmatism that might confound the observations. When the data were pooled, these individuals were found to have a minor but demonstrable deficit for seeing vertically oriented lines, just as predicted.

PLASTICITY IN THE ADULT CORTEX

The "deprivation rearing" experiments just described are just examples of a large body of similar research. A consistent finding of these studies is that the deprivation must occur very early in the life of the animal, in what is called the *critical period*. For example, the critical period in cats for monocular deprivation or horizontal/vertical rearing is the first few postnatal months. This limited period of sensitivity can be demonstrated by taking an older juvenile cat or an adult and sewing the lids of one eye shut or having them wear the special goggles for many months. When the eye is opened or the goggles are removed, the animal is found to be visually normal when tested behaviorally. Similarly, recording from its neurons in the visual cortex shows no deficits of the kinds just described for visually deprived kittens.

Thus, the common wisdom came to be that significant plasticity in sensory systems was only present at birth. Adult organisms were thought to have reached a point of stable, final wiring that could not be affected by any changes in their inputs. However, experiments over the last 15 years showed that such stability is not exactly the case. When looked for carefully, some plastic reorganization of adult sensory cortical areas does occur.

The next figure shows a prototypical example of such adult plasticity. A monkey's hand and its normal representation in the somatotopic map of a region of the primary somatosensory cortex (S1) are shown.

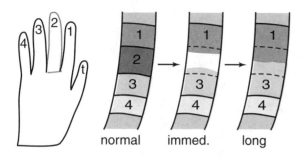

normal   immed.   long

there is still some plasticity based on sprouting of new axonal branches in the adult cortex.

Note, as discussed in earlier lectures, that each finger projects to an adjacent patch of cortex (*normal*). The blue line across the bottom of finger 2 indicates that the nerves to and from that finger that communicate with the cortex have been cut. Behaviorally, the animal immediately loses all sensation in the finger. Individual neurons in the region of the somatosensory cortex to which finger 2 projected were immediately recorded from, using microelectrodes. As expected, most of the neurons in that region are now silent (*indicated by the white patch*). However, at the margins of the region that normally responds to finger 2, the neurons now respond to the adjacent finger (*3 at the lower margin, 1 at the upper margin*). These new responses in region 2 are depicted by the "bleeding over" into region 2 of the colors representing regions *1* and *3*. The fact that the spreading of effective stimulation into the denervated patch of cortex occurs immediately is strong evidence that it is not a result of sprouting or any other kind of plasticity. Instead, it is probably due to synapses that were already present but were silenced by lateral inhibition when there was normal input to the region corresponding to finger 2.

The result of recordings from the cortex about a month after the denervation surgery holds the true surprise. The filling in of the colors (*right-most picture*) into the previously white region represents the finding that the cells that normally received inputs from finger 2 now are innervated by fingers 1 and 3. Anatomic examination shows that the responses are due to sprouting of axonal terminals from inputs related to fingers 1 and 3 into the newly opened up territory that previously "belonged" to finger 2. Such sprouting would be expected in a newborn animal. Its occurrence in a mature, adult animal was totally unexpected. The key point made by such results, which have been replicated in the other sensory areas of the cortex, is that

Interlude—*Musicians' Fingers*

Neuroimaging studies have been used to look at the cortical representation of the fingers of the left hand of adult professional violin players and of non-musicians. This is the hand that presses the strings to make all the notes, a task that requires speed and precision. The studies showed that the musicians had a larger amount of sensory cortex devoted to these fingers than do typical adults who do not play an instrument. Further, the degree of enlargement was positively correlated with the number of years an individual had played the violin. This result strongly supports the idea that very high usage leads to a plasticity-based spreading of the inputs from these fingers. Such an increase would be useful because the greater number of neurons in the enlarged areas, relative to normal, would lead to increased positional sensitivity of placement of the fingers during playing.

These findings strongly suggest that plastic changes in the sensory regions of adult brains are ongoing throughout adulthood, providing a basis for sharpening senses that are heavily used. Even more exciting, the finding of such plasticity suggests that carefully designed rehabilitation exercises might assist in reducing the effects of damage to neural pathways due to injury or strokes.

How much adult plasticity is there? Given the difficulty in proving the existence of such plasticity in adults, clearly, it is not as prevalent as in babies. Also, the degree of adult plasticity may turn out to vary in different systems (such as touch versus vision) or in the same system when it suffers various kinds of sensory "insults." However, the adult brain retains the ability to rewire in response to environmental changes to a degree that earlier studies suggested was not possible. An obvious and important question is whether the adult changes just discussed are carried out by cellular mechanisms that are the same as those that are the basis of learning and memory. Current research points to many similarities, but all of the evidence is far from in.

BEING

REVIEW

The previous lecture dealt with changes in the brain that are the basis of learning, memory, and synaptic restructuring after injury. It is very likely that many of the same basic cellular processes are involved in all of these long-lasting changes in the connections between neurons.

Memory is conceptualized into subtypes. Declarative memory consists of recall that is available to consciousness. Episodic memory contains entire scenes in which a particular memory was formed. Semantic memory consists of individual facts not tied to a particular episodic scene. Procedural memory typically does not involve conscious recall, but instead is linked to motor tasks, like riding a bicycle. Implicit memory is formed without any awareness that learning is occurring.

The hippocampus is fundamental to the processes that consolidate immediate and current memories (including working memories) into long-term memories that are stored in the temporal and frontal cortices. Memory storage is based on long-lasting changes in neuronal interactions. Much remains to be learned about the way this happens, and current

models postulate changes in the number and strength of synapses. Thus, polyneuronal circuits and their patterns of firing when stimulated would be the substrate of individual memories. At the molecular level, a possible model for such changes is the phenomenon of long-term potentiation (LTP). LTP is a process in which initial, intense activation of a synapse makes it more likely to become activated in response to subsequent stimulation, even days later. One way this happens is by the recruitment and insertion of new neurotransmitter receptors into the postsynaptic, dendritic side of a synapse.

Especially during early postnatal development, connections between neurons change as a result of experience, a process called neuronal plasticity. Although early postnatal plasticity has been recognized for about 50 years, new findings demonstrate that there is significant plasticity in the adult human cortex. Reorganization occurring due to repeated experience or after brain injuries is based on such adult plasticity. Deeper understanding of the mechanisms of plasticity will lead to useful therapeutic approaches in rehabilitation after injury or stroke.

What do these words have in common: *awake, asleep, conscious, unconscious*? They are all used to refer to a particular state of being. But, does the word *conscious* really belong on the list—is it really a "state of being"? Obviously, it belongs in the trivial sense of being the opposite of "knocked unconscious." However, when we say that Harry is conscious of the taste of his food, does *conscious* still have the same meaning? Probably not. When we say that Harry is *conscious of* something, we are implying that there is some inner state in his brain that he is aware of. But, how do

we know this "inner state" exists? And, do such inner states exist for animals?

For most of the twentieth century, neuroscientists avoided using the word *consciousness* and did not consider it a subject worthy of serious study, mainly because of its inherent subjectivity. Instead, behaviorism held center stage. In its basic form, *behaviorism* posits that an organism is a "black box" that receives input and generates output in response. The experimenter's job then consisted of determining the causal relationships between inputs and outputs. To do so, it was not necessary to know about the contents of the "black box." Why? Because causal relationships are like physical laws. For a behaviorist a question such as, "Why did the man run?" is answered in terms of careful characterization of the immediate stimuli, and a logical analysis of how the stimuli generate a response. There is no basis for answering the question by analyzing or even proposing the existence of any intent the man might have had that led to running.

What has come to be called *cognitive neuroscience* supplanted behaviorism as researchers gained a deeper understanding of the complex functioning of the brain. Recognizing the vastness and intricacy of its interconnections gave pause to simple stimulus-response explanations. Further, the concept of information was coming to the fore as a way of characterizing intelligence. Thinking was now conceptualized as a process needed to manipulate information. Cognition replaced stimulus-response explanations when discussing human actions.

To understand what is meant by the term *cognition*, consider this story. Dale was walking down the hall and saw Robby, naked, through a slightly open door. Dale stopped and stared. A few minutes later Robby saw Dale on the stairs and wanted to know what time Dale was coming to dinner. So, Robby called out, "Excuse me, Dale!" Dale turned and blushed deeply. Question: Why did Dale blush?

A cognitive explanation says that Dale, feeling guilty for staring, assumed that Robby was angry over that event and was about to chew Dale out. Such an explanation suggests that people believe that there is a particular thought in the mind of another. Further, this concept, called "theory of mind," fundamentally depends on the idea of intent.

The change of approach from behaviorism to cognition is very appealing, perhaps even "commonsensical." But, we also know that all of Dale's behavior in the story above was caused by the activity of neurons—electrical activity that follows causal and physical laws. So, how can a neuron, or even a group of neurons, have a *conscious intent*? When talking about neurons, does it even make sense to use the word *conscious* to mean anything other than the opposite of *unconscious*? This lecture explores such questions. If you are expecting answers based on compelling evidence, stop reading now. Such answers do not exist; part of this lecture examines the question of whether satisfactory answers can ever exist.

QUALIA AND THE COLOR-BLIND PHYSIOLOGIST

One essence of this lecture is captured by a story about a hypothetical professor. Imagine that Professor Albus was born with a developmental defect that prevented the formation of cones in her retina, which thus has only rod photoreceptors, a rare (but real) condition known as *rod monochromacy*. The word *monochromacy* characterizes the fact that such a person cannot discriminate among colors but only between shades of gray. In common parlance, a rod monochromat is totally color-blind and only sees in the black and white tones of old movies.

Wondering what the fuss about color is all about, Professor Albus recruits a normally sighted volunteer. She has some remarkable new technology. It allows her to noninvasively record lots of neurons in the volunteer's brain while he looks at visual stimuli. She also has a bunch of filters with different names on them, such as *red* and *green*. She puts one into a projector, flashes it for a second, and the subject says "red." At the same time she records a very detailed pattern of firing of neurons throughout the subject's visual cortex. When the filter labeled green is used, the subject says "green" and a different, highly specific pattern is recorded. Numerous repetitions lead Professor Albus to reliably differentiate between the patterns of neuronal activity generated by the red and green stimuli.

Next, an assistant puts one of the slides in the projector without Professor Albus knowing which it is. It is flashed on the screen. The subject sees it but says nothing. Professor Albus looks at the subject's pattern of action potentials and says, "Oh, that is green." In fact, by watching the action potential patterns she can always correctly say "red" or "green" when the stimulus is shown to the subject.

Question: As she properly says "red" or "green," does Professor Albus know what red and green look like? I hope you answered, "Of course not, she only knows about and recognizes the pattern of action potentials!" Surely, even if you knew that the technology she used allowed her to record every action potential in the subject's head and that the computing power to deal with all that information was available, you would still say, "No." But ask yourself what information does the subject have other than all the action potentials in his head and the computations that are going on in his neural networks? If the experience of analyzing action potentials cannot let Professor Albus know what red looks like, how is it that the analysis of those action potentials by the brain of the subject lets the subject know?

Let us examine this further. We know that "red" starts as the transduction of photons into ionic movements in photoreceptors. This electrical activity ultimately results in action potentials and postsynaptic potentials throughout the nervous system. These signals are just voltage changes caused by the physical movement of real ions in aqueous solution. Indeed, everything going on in your brain is just ions and molecules moving and changing shape or position—prototypical physical processes. How do those physical processes become redness?

This story exemplifies a well-debated problem. Redness is a quality of light that you *perceive*. Sweet is another such basic quality, as are warmth and the particular odor of a fresh rose. In the jargon of philosophy (which likes to use words from ancient languages), redness, sweetness, and so on, are called *qualia*. (*Qualia* is the plural form; the singular is *quale*). Defined a bit more precisely, qualia are the fundamental sense perceptions that you have when particular stimuli assail you. Further, qualia are something you are aware of consciously: you know it when you see red.

Note that we are not asking another familiar question, namely, is what you perceive when you see red the same as what I perceive when I see red? I do not know, or even know how I could know. But we have come to a cultural agreement to call it red. The question being asking is, "What *is* redness?" Or, to put it in physical terms, how does the movement of sodium and potassium and a few other ions in your brain become redness?

The question of how the brain makes qualia is part of an age-old philosophical discussion known as the "mind/brain problem." This problem asks the question, "How does brain make mind?" The philosopher David Chalmers recently brought the issue of how neural activity becomes qualia once again to the forefront of consciousness studies. He calls it "the hard question." He does so to differentiate between the hard question and other questions such as, how do we recognize faces, or how do we direct attention to a particular thing, or what is the physical basis of a memory? Chalmers claims that the kind of explanations given throughout this book answer the latter questions, or will do so in the foreseeable future. However, he and many others assert that the hard question will not, perhaps even cannot, be answered in physiologic terms.

DUELING WITH DUALISTS

Possibly you might be saying about now, "Are not qualia and thoughts different from the *physical* stuff that goes on in the brain? Isn't a thought or the sensation of qualia a *mental* thing?" The idea that there are physical and mental activities that occur in the brain, and that they are different, is called *dualism*. The idea was most famously put forward in the 1600s by Descartes, with his famous statement, "*Cogito ergo sum*," which translates to, "I think, therefore I am." He meant to distinguish between the base, animal-like machine that was his physical body and the "I" that was the higher, mental, thinking part.

You might reasonably state the criticism that dualism answers the hard question by ignoring it and instead makes up a state of being called "mental" that is different from physical. Indeed, dualism has been severely maligned in the past hundred years, and currently, few philosophers or physiologists claim to support it as a reasonable position.

What do they offer instead? In one form or another, their reply is that mind is nothing more than the working of the brain. A classy way of rephrasing this position is to say, "The brain is the organ of the mind." Mind happens because the brain is working in the same sense that circulation happens because the heart is pumping or that digestion happens because the stomach and intestines are functioning.

The critics of dualism, sometimes labeled *reductionists*, say that today we do not know enough about how the brain works to know how it "makes" mind. But, they say, one day we will, and that is that, so just be patient, stop useless philosophizing, and keep plugging away on understanding how the brain works. When we know enough, the hard question will evaporate.

Interlude—*Nothing Else Is in There*

The following well-known thought experiment is used to argue that dualism cannot be right because nothing else is "in there."

We can implant artificial hips when necessary. Even artificial hearts have been implanted, although they do not yet work as well as a real one. Prosthetic devices are getting better and better. Imagine that in the wonderful future we are able to make prosthetic axons that carry out the same function as real ones, although they are not made out of membranes and cytoplasm. We learn how to attach them between cell bodies and boutons, curing multiple sclerosis and spinal cord injuries. "Far-fetched," you say? Sure, but this Interlude *is* a thought experiment and there is nothing technical that might prevent the development of such prosthetic axons.

Now, the big question: If all the axons in your body were replaced by prosthetic ones, would your mind or your consciousness cease to exist? "No," is the common answer. In principle, axon replacement is not different from hip replacement, and that replacement does not make anyone less human. Let's go on. The mature, neuronal cell body is basically a bag of metabolic reactions. As we come to know more and more about these, eventually we could develop a prosthetic soma. So, if in addition to the axons we now replace all of your neuronal cell bodies with prosthetic ones, would your mind or your consciousness cease to exist? If you agreed the answer above is "No," then there is no reason to answer differently here. By now you see where this line of reasoning is going: with prosthetic dendrites and prosthetic synapses, eventually nothing original is left in your cranium. And each time, the answer to the question, "Would the mind cease to exist?" is "No."

Wait a minute! Our thought experiment has replaced every part of the cellular neuronal circuitry of the brain with prosthetic, physical devices of known function. There is nothing "mental" about any of the physical replacement apparatus. It is all just well-engineered "stuff." So, on what basis could a dualist say that there is something else in there?

In fairness, we must mention still another position, one that is currently most identified with the philosopher Daniel Dennett. Simply put, he says that qualia, mind, and consciousness do not exist. (He argues more elegantly than such a brief restatement of his position implies.) He takes the position that these are words we invent to describe things we do not understand, similar in concept to the "tooth fairy." While this position could be true, the rest of this lecture is based on the assumption (and your daily personal experience) that qualia and consciousness do exist.

CAN WE KNOW?

Is it possible that the experience of consciousness is real but that we simply cannot prove that it is? Gödel's theorem is often brought up in support of the idea that we cannot prove the existence of consciousness. Gödel proved analytically than no mathematical system that is logically complete (e.g., euclidean geometry) can be used to prove its own axioms, even if they are true. In colloquial terms, Gödel's theorem can be restated to say that we cannot use the brain to understand the brain itself. Such an application of Gödel's theorem sounds good, but it depends on agreeing that "understanding the brain" is equivalent to "a formal logical system." Some agree, some do not.

If Gödel's theorem tells us that we cannot expect mathematics to help us, what about using language? The philosopher Benson Mates argues that language will not work either. He starts by observing that we never really know the exact truth but only know what our limited intellect and technology can tell us about it. Namely, human knowledge has fundamental, built-in limitations. One such limitation is the nature of language itself, which has unresolvable, intrinsic ambiguities. Mates uses the well-known "liar's paradox" to illustrate such ambiguity.

The paradox, first recorded by Greek philosophers over 3000 years ago, is whether or not to believe a person who says, "Everything I say is false." What is paradoxical about this? Well, if the statement is true, then it tells us that it itself must be false, in which case it cannot be true. On the other hand, if its false, that says that the opposite, "Everything I say is true," is true, but that must mean that the statement "Everything I say is false," is true. It almost hurts to think about it, doesn't it? But there is no way out. Our language, which reflects our way of thought, simply is intrinsically ambiguous at times. Mates suggests that statements like the liar's paradox, called *antinomies*, are analogous to the impossibility of understanding consciousness using language as a medium of explanation and understanding.

WHAT ARE THE CHARACTERISTICS OF CONSCIOUSNESS?

If we are to learn anything about consciousness, we must first characterize what we mean when we use the word. Even if trying to nail down the meaning of the concept of consciousness does not provide an answer to the hard question, it might shed some light on where to look and how to do the looking. It might even provide categories of behavior that can be studied by fMRI. At the least, such research could let us know what the brain is doing when consciousness occurs.

A good way to proceed is to try to list attributes of consciousness. Here are some that have been proposed:

- *Awareness,* sometimes described as an ability to perceive elements of the external environment. (A difference between awareness and awakeness can be captured by the assertion that one must be awake to be aware, but one does not need to be aware to be awake.)
- *Self-awareness,* a sense of "I-ness," including sensations of qualities like the redness of a light or the painness of pain. Sensory maps of various bodily spaces seem to be in this category as well.
- *Temporality,* a sense of nowness and of time, including a sense of the past and future.
- *Memory,* related to temporality but not the same. Imagine an animal that sees a stick, remembers "stick," and equates it with "pain" because it was once hit by a stick; however, it does not have any history in its mind of when that happened relative to other events.
- *Feelings,* including emotions and desires.
- *Intentions* and *expectations.*
- *Thoughts*, including beliefs, ideas, manipulation of symbols, reasoning, and inner imagery.

Coming from a different starting point, the philosopher Ned Block proposed different "kinds" of consciousness, in his article titled "Consciousness" in the book *A Companion to the Philosophy of Mind*:

- *Phenomenal consciousness*: The way things seem to us; the way pain feels; experiential qualities of sensation.
- *Self-consciousness*: "The possession of a concept of the self and the ability to use this concept in thinking about oneself. . . . There is reason to believe that animals or babies can have phenomenally conscious states without employing any concept of self."
- *Monitoring consciousness*: A conscious state ". . . that is accompanied by a thought to the effect that one is in that state. . . . Dogs and babies may have phenomenally conscious pains without thoughts to the effect that they have those pains."
- *Access-consciousness*: "A state is access-conscious if, in virtue of one's having the state, a representation of its content is (a) . . . freely available as a premise in reasoning, and (b) poised for rational control of action, and (c) poised for rational control of speech."

WHO IS ME?

Let's try to use one of these distinctions, self-consciousness, to return to the study of brain physiology. First, we need to describe what is generally meant when the term *self* is used by cognitive scientists. We use the word *describe*, rather than *define*, because the concept of self is as slippery as consciousness. Some of the attributes of self include

- Experience of ownership
- Long-term unity of beliefs
- Continuity of experience
- Center of spatial awareness and body sense
- Subject of extended narrative
- Locus of memories and experience
- Differentiation from "other."

In putting forward such attributes, we do not mean to imply that the "self" is a separate little person inside the head who is the watcher of all that happens. Such a dualistic, Cartesian view gets us nowhere in trying to understand what it is about the brain that generates a sense of self. Similarly, looking for one particular part of the brain that represents the self with neuroimaging techniques is likely to represent a failed modern form of dualism. In the end, probably all of the attributes listed above, and more, add up to a subjective inner experience called self that is in the same category of subjective experience as qualia. Further, self is likely to be the essence of a parallel process, with many diffuse brain networks contributing to it.

Looking at the list of attributes of self, we can make a start at relating them to the brain by noting that the physical sense of self in space has already been revealed by the condition of parietal hemineglect discussed in Lecture 4. Recall that patients with a certain kind of right parietal lobe lesion lose any sense of the existence of the left side of their bodies. Thus, activity in the right parietal association area must be part of the process that is self. Areas of the frontal lobe that are related to recognizing that a memory is a memory, and not a new event being perceived, must also play a role. Recent work also implicates a frontal locus in the process of differentiating self from other.

THE MIRROR TEST

An aspect of knowing that "I am a self" is captured by my realization that the image I see when I look in a mirror is me. A typical child does not have such self-recognition until about the age of 2. Among the primates, only a few of the great apes display self-recognition, and some experiments argue that dolphins also do. How is such self-recognition determined in these animals? For apes, a spot of white dust is surreptitiously painted on an animal's forehead. Sometime later the animal is allowed to look in a mirror. The question is, does the animal behave as if the image in the mirror is another ape, or is the image recognized as self? If the image is thought to be another, we might expect that the animal doing the looking realizes that the ape represented by the mirror has some funny dirt on its forehead. Grooming behavior would take over and the real ape would pick at the mirror, trying to get the dirt off the "other" ape. However, if the ape realizes it is looking at itself, it would reach to its own forehead (which it obviously cannot see directly) and brush off the white powder while looking in the mirror to guide its actions. Such self-grooming is exactly what many of the great apes do. In contrast, lower primates, such as rhesus monkeys, try to groom the mirror.

THEORY OF MIND

The distinction that *I* constitute a subject who is fundamentally different from *you* is the concept called "Theory of Mind" (TOM). Namely, I know that what is going on in your head is different from what is going on in mine, and I have theories about your thoughts. The story about Dale and Robby earlier in this lecture demonstrates TOM. The explanation only makes sense if we accept that the blush is a response to what Dale theorizes is in Robby's mind. A child under the age of 2

or 3 does not make such distinctions, and it is not until ages 6 to 8 that a child can recognize and explain complex stories based on a well-formed TOM.

Interpreting verbal stories based on TOM proved to be an interesting way to look for brain activity related to self-versus-other. Experimenters asked subjects to read stories while being scanned with MRI. After each presentation they were then asked a question that required them to interpret what they read. Subjects did not respond verbally but only thought about the answer. Some of the stories and pictures were of the Dale/Robby type. Thus, when the subjects thought about their answers, they needed to use an internalized TOM. Other stories and pictures did not require such interpretations but only the application of logic (e.g., "While John was running he unexpectedly stubbed his toe on a rock and fell." Question: "Why did John fall?"). When the fMRI data derived from the non-TOM-type stimuli were subtracted from the fMRI data recorded during thinking that required use of a TOM, an area in the frontal cortex was found to be selectively activated by the TOM tasks.

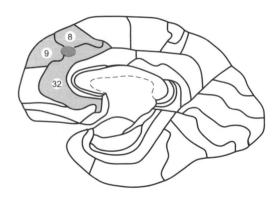

The activated area is shown schematically by the blue oval at the approximate boundaries of Brodmann areas 8, 9, and 32 in this picture of the medial surface of the right hemisphere. Similar locations in both the left and right hemispheres were simultaneously active. No claim is made that the activated region is the "seat of the mind" or even the location where the TOM is stored. However, the result does validate the concept that a TOM exists.

Adults who suffer from the mental condition known as *autism* have a great deal of trouble relating to other people and when asked to interpret stories, do poorly on TOM tests. *Asperger's syndrome* is a mild form of autism. People with Asperger's syndrome also have difficulty with TOM tests. A group of such subjects was studied with MRI using TOM tests similar to those just described. No task-related activity was found in the frontal area shown in the diagram, further strengthening the idea that TOM relates to specific processes that occur in the frontal lobe.

Interlude—*Multiple Minds?*

The condition called *multiple personality disorder* (MPD) has captured the attention of audiences of movies, TV programs, and numerous magazine articles. The defense that "my other self did it" has even been offered in criminal trials. Do such people really have multiple personalities, or are they just making up alternate personas for some reason? How might one brain have multiple "selves"?

The reality of MPD has been debated at length in the psychiatric literature for decades. Some accept it as a variant form of schizophrenia; others say such people are fooling themselves and us with a complex story. If MPD does exist, what could be a brain-related explanation? Maintaining a long-term self requires binding together a myriad of memories and present experiences. It is possible that cortical association areas are malfunctioning in persons with MPD, thus keeping them from coalescing their memories and experiences. Such malfunction could be analogous to the way in which schizophrenics who hear a voice do not know the voice is really them, as discussed in Lecture 7.

Can modern neuroimaging techniques provide evidence of the reality of MPD? A recent finding is very suggestive. A female patient with two personalities was studied using fMRI during the moments of switching from her main personality to her alter personality, and back. (She could make the switches voluntarily when asked.) The fMRI studies showed that hippocampal and medial temporal areas were specifically inhibited during the switch, with the switch to the alternate personality involving mainly the left hippocampus and the switch back the right hippocampus. The temporal areas involved were ones where memory processes normally occur. There are too many ways to interpret this study to allow firm conclusions. However, it suggests that something more than play acting is going on.

DREAMING: ALTERED CONSCIOUSNESS

It is reasonable to consider dreaming as being an altered state of consciousness, in contrast to simple unconsciousness. For example, brain activity similar to awake activity occurs during dreams, but not in comatose unconsciousness. Thus, focusing on the differences between waking consciousness and dreaming consciousness might help our quest for understanding consciousness in general.

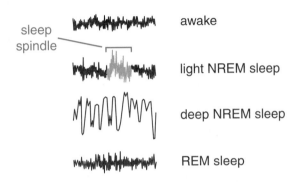

Sleep has a number of different stages that are easily monitored and identified by EEG recordings made using electrodes on the scalp. The stages are illustrated in the above figure, all to the same scale. The awake EEG is generally characterized by low-voltage desynchronized activity. As you start to fall asleep, you enter non-rapid-eye-movement (NREM) sleep, which has four levels, two of which are shown here. In light NREM sleep (stage 2) the EEG is a bit decreased in frequency and slightly larger in amplitude than when awake. Also, recognizable bursts, called *sleep spindles*, are characteristic of this stage. In deep NREM sleep (stage 4) the EEG becomes highly synchronized, slowed in frequency, and significantly increased in amplitude.

In a typical young adult it takes about 1 hour to reach NREM stage 4, which then lasts about another hour. It is then followed by rapid-eye-movement (REM) sleep, which is named for the fact that beneath the closed lids the eyes suddenly start to rapidly move back and forth. A key point is to notice that the EEG during REM sleep is very similar to the awake EEG and very different from the deep NREM EEG.

REM sleep is the period when vivid dreaming occurs. A different type of dreaming, more realistic in nature, happens during light NREM sleep. Here we focus on dreaming during REM sleep in the comparison with awake consciousness, mainly because the similarities and differences are striking. The following table is adapted from the book *Consciousness* by the sleep researcher J. Allan Hobson.

Parameter	Awake	REM Sleep
Sensory input	High	Low
Motor output	Strong	Blocked
Thought	Organized	Illogical
Insight	Good	Delusional
Memory—recent	Good	Poor
Memory—past	Good	Good

Three key points are illustrated. First, cognitive activity, exemplified here by thought and insight, occurs during both dreaming and the awake state. However, the controlled and organized cognitive activities of awake consciousness give way to delusional and fantastic cognition during dreaming. Second, the consciousness of dreaming is basically out of touch with the external world. Only the most vigorous external stimuli that might signify danger get through to the dreamer. Also, output is heavily inhibited. Muscle activity is almost paralyzed during REM dreaming, probably to keep the body from flailing about in reflexive response to the content of dreams. Third, there is access to memory in both states, but the ability to make new memories during dreaming is severely limited. Such memory impairment is why we can report a dream when awakened during it or shortly thereafter but otherwise have trouble remembering our dreams. Addressing these three points physiologically gives clues to the brain mechanisms related to consciousness.

THE RETICULAR FORMATION

We need to start with staying awake, which requires an understanding of the reticular formation. *Reticulum* is the name used for a loosely interconnected, functionally related collection of neurons whose cell bodies are not grouped near each other. (*Reticulum* contrasts with the word *nucleus*, which is used in naming a

tightly compact group of neurons, as in the *dentate nucleus*.) Typically a reticulum is tangled around many nuclei and integrates a large number of diverse inputs that arise in those nuclei.

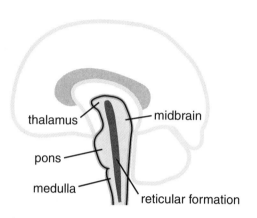

A specific example is the brainstem reticular formation. As shown in this figure, it is a sausage-shaped grouping of neurons that runs up the core of the brainstem from the medulla to the thalamus. It is actually a set of paired structures, although only the right member of the pair is depicted here in this medial view of the right hemisphere.

Neurons in the reticular formation are in the perfect position to integrate all of the sensory activity that is passing from the cortex to the spinal cord and the body. So, a reticular neuron does not have the specificity to know what sounds are coming from the cochlea, but can reflect the overall degree of auditory activity. In fact, reticular formation cells usually are polysensory, adding up many aspects of sensory input. (You might imagine such a neuron, if it could speak, saying, "Wow it is noisy and bright out there!")

A key component of the reticular formation is the *reticular activating system* (RAS). The RAS is a collection of neurons that lie mainly in the pontine part of the reticular formation and that use acetylcholine as their neurotransmitter. These neurons have long axons that project to other brainstem areas, the thalamus, and many cortical areas, especially the basal forebrain. The RAS is called an "activating system" because its activity is necessary for maintaining wakefulness. A significant decrease of RAS activity is a major cause of the NREM sleep stages. In contrast, the RAS is hyperactive during REM sleep, a situation reflected in the similarity of the awake EEG and the REM sleep EEG patterns.

This dream state arousal also activates the neuronal firing that contributes to dreaming by internal stimulation of the visual system, and other cortical sensory areas and emotional systems. We can thus generalize to say that consciousness requires an active process of stimulation that arises mainly from the cholinergic RAS.

If the RAS is active, why are not you awake during REM sleep? The answer lies in the behavior during sleep of other reticular formation subsystems. For example, there is a set of neurons that turns down motor output, resulting in the near paralysis that occurs during REM sleep. Two other major systems in the reticular formation, the serotonin and the norepinephrine projection systems, are turned down during sleep. Both of these project widely to the cortex, where their outputs are normally responsible for activating and focusing attention and allowing the formation of memory. Because these systems are "off" during REM sleep, key neural circuits are inhibited. These include those that focus on important aspects of stimuli, that compare intent with result, that remember in the short term what came before what (and that allow long-term memories to form), and that correlate emotions with actions. Thus, REM sleep cognition loses various aspects of internal coordination, leading to the fantastic and bizarre nature of dreams.

To generalize, the sensible nature of cognition that we call waking consciousness is an active process. Consciousness requires that numerous networks throughout the cortex actively communicate and work with each other. Put in other words, consciousness does not just happen; it takes work to be conscious!

WHAT IS CONSCIOUSNESS GOOD FOR?

If we make the reasonable assumption that human self-consciousness evolved when our primate ancestors evolved all of the other features that eventually led to *Homo sapiens*, the question can be asked, "What do you get with consciousness that is advantageous—what was selected for?" Speculation and opinion predominate answers to this question but still lend insight into ways that the brain and world interact. Also, it is useful to expand the question a bit by including human language in our answers because language

is a primary component of the expression of our consciousness.

Conscious thought allows for complex and flexible social understanding. There can be an "I" and a "you" who interact socially only because I can distinguish *self* from *other*. Further, I understand your intentions and motives because I have introspective access to the intentions and motives of my behavior. "I know what you are thinking," really means, "I know what I would be thinking in this situation." Also, my self-knowledge gives me a benchmark against which to judge you, perhaps when I'm deciding on your fitness as a possible mate.

Human consciousness allows us to express the concept of past and future in concrete terms. It lets us plan, based on experience, and to have organized behavior with long-term goals. For example, I can tell you a story about what I plan to do next week and how I plan to do it when I go hunting. Based on the story, you can decide if you want to wait here and then go with me or to leave now. Think how hard it would be to negotiate such a future partnership, which might be important to survival, without consciousness expressed through language. Consciousness lets me tell an imaginary story as if it was a fact and to plan according to my evaluation of that fiction.

Finally, consciousness allows complex social interactions because it allows us to assign moral implications to actions. We can develop concepts such as guilt and altruism that can guide and govern our behavior, rather than simply respond to instinctual emotional drives. As a result, society can go beyond grooming, mating, and simple survival.

OF ASPIRIN AND ELEPHANTS: WILL WE EVER UNDERSTAND CONSCIOUSNESS?

I am not the first to suggest that something fundamental may be missing when many intelligent people study the same problem and come up with numerous conflicting and unsatisfying explanations. As an example, consider the common drug aspirin. Prior to the middle of the twentieth century there were numerous, conflicting scientific papers that purported to explain how aspirin lowers fever, none of them satisfactory. At that time, no one had yet discovered how a group of hormone-like substances called *prostaglandins* function. Now we know that aspirin works in part by interacting with the prostaglandins. The large number of conflicting papers about how aspirin works reflected the fact that something fundamental—prostaglandins and their function—remained to be discovered.

We appear to be in a similar situation regarding the study of consciousness. There are numerous ferociously held theories about what consciousness is. Worse, some theories say consciousness isn't—that it simply cannot or does not exist. This morass of ideas is put forward by intelligent people who have carefully considered the subject. Yet their disagreements are often extreme. When reading their criticisms of each other, I wonder how each can claim the other is so wrongheaded. Why can't they understand each other's arguments and agree on some logically consistent conclusion?

Is consciousness like aspirin? Will someone ever discover the consciousness equivalent of the prostaglandins that lets us jump out of all our incomplete and imperfect thinking? Perhaps, and then again perhaps not. Consider the old story of the blind people and the elephant. Recall that one touched the trunk, one the tail, one a leg, one the side of the body, one a soft floppy ear, and one a firm tusk. Each gave a description of the wondrous creature that differed wildly from the others. Because of their limited perceptions, they were unable to grasp a fundamental unity in what they individually perceived. Perhaps with the input of different information from a newly sighted person, they could have put the elephant together again. And, maybe consciousness will yield to our understanding in some similar fashion.

Or, we may be destined to never know. Imagine a group of two-dimensional, sighted persons who live in a two-dimensional plane that is embedded in a three-dimensional world. That is, they experience their world as an infinitely thin sheet of paper, which a famous book that explores it calls "Flatland." Now, imagine further that Flatland exists on a single, unmovable plane that goes exactly through the middle of a three-dimensional elephant. Each Flatlander perceives a part of the two-dimensional outline of part of the elephant. However, even if the Flatlanders get together and pool all their data, they will never understand the three-dimensional elephant. Here, the something fundamental that is missing is a dimension that they can never discover, given the limitations of their existence. But, it's fun trying!

APPENDIX I: Names and Places

This list uses a standardized hierarchy and names adopted by the *BrainInfo* database at <http://braininfo.rprc.washington.edu/mainmenu.html>.

HINDBRAIN
Medulla oblongata
Cochlear nuclei
Medullary reticular formation
Solitary nucleus
Inferior olivary complex
Vestibular nuclei
Metencephalon
Cerebellum
Deep cerebellar nuclei
Dentate nucleus
Fastigial nucleus
Globose nucleus
Emboliform nucleus
Cerebellar cortex
Flocculonodular lobe
Posterior lobe
Vermis of posterior lobe
Anterior lobe
Pons
Basal part of pons
Pontine nuclei
Pontine tegmentum
Pontine reticular formation
Superior olivary complex
Locus ceruleus

MIDBRAIN
Cerebral Peduncle
Substantia nigra
Midbrain tegmentum
Midbrain reticular formation
Red nucleus
Oculomotor nuclei
Tectum
Inferior colliculus
Superior colliculus
Pretectal region

FOREBRAIN
Diencephalon
Subthalamus
Zona incerta
Subthalamic nucleus
Hypothalamus
Intermediate hypothalamic region
Hypophysis
Adenohypophysis
Neurohypophysis
Thalamus
Metathalamus
Medial geniculate body
Lateral geniculate body
Epithalamus
Habenula
Pineal body
Telencephalon
Cerebral cortex
Archicortex
Hippocampal formation
Hippocampus
Dentate gyrus
Subiculum
Parahippocampal gyrus
Cingulate gyrus
Occipital lobe
Temporal lobe
Insula
Parietal lobe
Frontal lobe
Cerebral white matter
Anterior commissure
Internal capsule
Corpus callosum
Basal ganglia
Amygdala
Globus pallidus
Striatum
Caudate nucleus
Putamen
Septum
Fornix
Olfactory bulb

Divisions of the Brain		
Embryonic	Adult	Components
Prosencephalon (forebrain)	Telencephalon (endbrain)	Cerebral cortex Basal ganglia Limbic system Hippocampus
	Diencephalon (interbrain)	Thalamus Hypothalamus
Mesencephalon (midbrain)		Tectum Tegmentum
Rhombencephalon (hindbrain)	Metencephalon	Cerebellum Pons Tegmentum
	Myelencephalon	Medulla oblongata

This table lists divisions and commonly used names of brain regions. The forebrain, midbrain, and hindbrain are physically separate regions during the development of the human embryo, and two of them give rise to two subdivisions that are distinct in the adult. Thus, there are five divisions. Starting at the top of the head and going down to the spinal cord, they are the telencephalon, diencephalon, mesencephalon, metencephalon, and myelencephalon. Each has homologs in the brains of lower animals. The earliest brains are all hindbrains, more advanced animals added a midbrain, and the cerebral cortex comes into its own mainly in mammals.

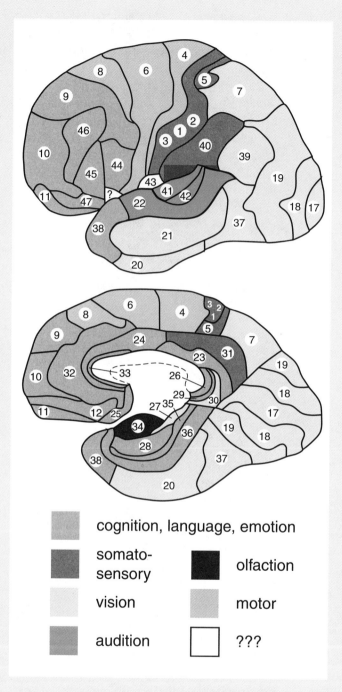

cognition, language, emotion

somato-sensory   olfaction

vision   motor

audition   ???

Brodmann's areas as defined in his 1909 publication. Numbers "missing" in this sequence only exist in his maps of monkey cortex. The attributions of function have been developed since his anatomic descriptions. The functions identified here are not as subdivided as the ones in the pictures throughout this book, in the interests of keeping this diagram clear and simple.

APPENDIX II: *Terms for Cognitive, Behavioral, and Neurologic Disorders*

This is a comprehensive list of terms used to describe altered states associated with brain injury such as trauma, stroke, or tumor or with developmental deficits. Most psychiatric diagnostic terms (e.g., schizophrenia), disease names, and named syndromes are not included.

Related forms vary in starting with the prefix *a-*, *dys-*, or *para-*. Words beginning *a-* signify a *complete* absence, lack, or inability; i.e., *aphagia* is the inability to swallow. Words beginning with *dys-* signify *partial* loss or disability; i.e., *dysphagia* is difficulty swallowing. The *para-* form is a generalization meaning *abnormal*. These prefix conventions are not always followed rigorously. All commonly used forms are listed (and cross-referenced in brackets) for ease of use of this list.

The following definitions are paraphrased from definitions in a large number of print and on-line dictionaries, and neurology textbooks.

Abasia (dysbasia): Inability to walk properly, taking steps that are too big or too small.
Ablepsia: Blindness.
Abulia: Loss of willpower or ability to make decisions.
Acalculia (dyscalculia, anarithmetria): Inability to use mathematics.
Acataphasia: Inability to formulate a statement or expression in an organized manner.
Achromatopsia: Complete color blindness; able only to see shades of black and white.
Acoria (akoria): Inability to feel satiated, regardless of how much is eaten.
Acyanopsia (tritanopia): Color blindness in the blue region of the spectrum.
Adiadochokinesia (dysdiadochokinesia): Inability to perform rapidly alternating movements, that is, to stop a movement and follow it with another in an opposite direction.
Ageusia (parageusia, ageustia): Loss of the sense of taste.
Ageustia (ageusia, parageusia): Loss of the sense of taste.
Agnosia: A general term for a loss of ability to recognize objects, people, sounds, shapes, or smells; that is, an inability to attach meaning to objective sense-data. Usually used when the primary sense organ involved is not impaired.
Agraphesthesia: Inability to identify a letter or number being written on a part of the body.
Agraphia (dysgraphia): Inability to express thought in written language (usually not due to mechanical dysfunction).
Agrypnia (ahypnia): Insomnia.
Ahypnia (agrypnia): Insomnia.
Akathisia: Motor restlessness; an inability to sit still. Often caused by defects in the extrapyramidal system.
Akinesia (dyskinesia, parakinesia): Extreme reluctance to perform elementary motor activities. A form of apraxia.
Akoria (acoria): Inability to feel satiated, regardless of how much is eaten.
Alalia: Inability to speak.
Alexia: Inability to read and understand written language. A subform of dyslexia.
Allesthesia: Perception of the limb opposite to the one stimulated. Related to dyschiria.
Alliesthesia: Perception of the same external stimulus as sometimes pleasant and sometimes unpleasant.
Allodynia: Pain caused by a normally nonpainful stimulus.
Allolalia: Speech disorder.
Alogia: Speech defect due to a brain lesion or injury.
Amelodia (aprosodia): Absence of normal variations of pitch, rhythm, and stress in speech.
Amentia: Extreme mental retardation.
Amnesia: Total or partial loss of memory.
Amusia: Inability to produce or appreciate musical sounds.
Anacusia: Deafness.
Analgesia: Absence of a normal sense of pain.
Anarithmetria (acalculia, dyscalculia): Inability to use mathematics.
Anarthria: A general term related to altered speech that includes either aphonia or aprosodia.

Anergia: Listless or lacking in energy.

Anhedonia: Inability to experience pleasure.

Anomia (dysnomia): General term for the inability to name objects. Can be limited to objects in semantic categories such as living things, inanimate things, fruits, colors, etc.

Anopsia: Blindness in one eye.

Anorexia (dysorexia): Loss of appetite as part of a pathologic fear of weight gain.

Anosmia (dysosmia, anosphrasia): Lack of the sense of smell.

Anosognosia: Unawareness of, denial of, or failure to recognize one's own neurologic deficit. For example, people paralyzed on the left side may claim an ability to move their left arm.

Anosphrasia (anosmia, dysosmia): Loss of sense of smell.

Apastia: Refusal to eat.

Aphagia (dysphagia): Difficulty swallowing.

Aphasia (dysphasia): General term that literally means "no speech." It refers to any impairment of the ability to use or understand words and can be used to describe loss of one or more of the following: ability to speak, ability to write, ability to understand speech, ability to understand written words. Major subcategories include *Broca's aphasia*, in which one can comprehend speech but not produce it, and *Wernicke's aphasia* in which one can produce speech but not comprehend it.

Aphemia: Inability to speak words but able to make other sounds.

Aphonia (dysphonia): Loss of ability to speak; inability to produce speech sounds. Distinguished from the motor defect dysarthria.

Aphrasia: Inability to make intelligible spoken sentences.

Apraxia (dyspraxia): Difficulty in performing a learned movement or coordinated motor activity even though understanding, motor coordination, and sensation are normal. Specific apraxias may be limited to a certain group of functions, such as inability to dress oneself.

Aprosodia (amelodia): Absence of normal variations of pitch, rhythm, and stress in speech.

Areflexia (dysreflexia): Absent reflex in response to a stimulus.

Asemia: Loss of ability to express or understand symbols or signs of thought.

Asitia: Lack of appetite or loathing of food.

Astasis: Inability to stand due to lack of motor coordination but having normal strength.

Astereognosia: Inability to identify objects that are palpated.

Asthenia: General weakness or debilitation.

Asynergia: Loss of motor coordination.

Ataxia: Poor coordination and unsteadiness due to failure to regulate the body's posture, and strength and direction of limb movements.

Atonia: Lack of muscle tension or tone.

Bradykinesia: Abnormal slowness of movement caused by a neurologic defect.

Circumlocution: Evasive speech or use of unusual definitions.

Confabulation: Answering of questions by an inappropriate, made-up attempt to explain.

Coprolalia: Offensive speech such as swear words.

Déjà vu (paramnesia): The illusory experience that something was previously experienced but is actually being experienced for the first time.

Dementia: General term for loss of intellectual or cognitive abilities.

Deuteranopia: Color blindness in which bluish red and green are confused.

Diplopia: Double vision.

Dysacusis: Distortion of hearing of sound frequency or intensity, often painful.

Dysaesthesia (dysesthesia): Abnormal sensations of the skin. Sometimes used more generally for the impairment of any of the senses.

Dysantigraphia: Inability to copy writing or printed letters.

Dysaphia: Impaired sense of touch.

Dysarthria: Imperfect articulation of speech due to disturbances of muscular control. This is distinguished from aphonia.

Dysbasia (abasia): Difficulty walking, usually by taking steps that are too big or too small.

Dyscalculia (acalculia, anarithmetria): Impaired ability to use mathematics.

Dyschiria: Inability to tell which side of the body has been touched.

Dyschronation: Distorted sense of time.

Dysdiadochokinesia (adiadochokinesia): Difficulty in performing rapidly alternating movements, that is, to stop a movement and follow it with another in an opposite direction.

Dysergia: Motor impairment due to axonal transmission failure.

Dysesthesia (dysaesthesia): Abnormal sensations of the skin. Sometimes used more generally for the impairment of any of the senses.

Dysgraphia (agraphia): Difficulty expressing thought in written language (usually not due to mechanical dysfunction).

Dyskinesia (akinesia, parakinesia): Extreme reluctance to perform elementary motor activities. A form of apraxia.

Dyslexia: Difficulty in properly interpreting or producing written language. Individuals can see and recognize letters but have difficulty spelling and writing words. They have no impairment of intelligence, or of object or picture identification.

Dyslogia: Difficulty in expressing ideas.

Dysmetria: Uncoordinated movement that misses its target.

Dysmimia: Difficulty in expressing oneself by gestures or signs. Inability to physically imitate.

Dysmorphophobia: Obsession that a normal body part is malformed or poor in appearance.

Dysnomia (anomia): General term for a difficulty in naming objects. Can be limited to objects in semantic categories such as living things, inanimate things, fruits, colors, etc.

Dysorexia (anorexia): Loss of appetite as part of a pathologic fear of weight gain.

Dysosmia (anosmia, anosphrasia): Lack of the sense of smell.

Dysphagia (aphagia): Difficulty swallowing.

Dysphasia (aphasia): Impairment of the ability to use or understand words.

Dysphemia: Substitution of an offensive word for an ordinary one.

Dysphonia (aphonia): Impaired ability to speak or to produce speech sounds. Distinguished from the motor defect dysarthria.

Dyspraxia (apraxia): Difficulty in performing a learned movement or coordinated motor activity even though understanding, motor coordination, and sensation are normal. Specific dyspraxias may be limited to a certain group of functions, such as difficulty in dressing oneself.

Dysreflexia (areflexia): Abnormal reflex in response to a stimulus.

Dyssomnia: Disordered sleep such as insomnia or hypersomnia.

Dyssynergia: Disorganized motor movement.

Dystonia: Maintenance of a persistent posture or position; locked into position.

Echolalia: Imitation of sounds without comprehension of their meaning. Normal in children but an abnormality in adults.

Echopraxia: Involuntary imitation of the movements made by another.

Environmental agnosia: Inability to orient to physically familiar places but able to orient to an abstract representation such as a map.

Hemianopsia: Loss of either the left or right half of the field of vision.

Hemiballismus: Wild, involuntary movement of the limbs on one side of the body.

Hemiparesis: Muscle weakness on one side of the body.

Hemiplegia: Complete paralysis of one side of the body.

Hyperacusis: Extreme sensitivity to sounds.

Hyperalgesia (hyperpathia): Increased reaction to a stimulus, especially a repetitive stimulus, as well as an increased threshold. Often painful.

Hyperkinesia: Abnormal quickness of movement caused by a neurologic defect.

Hyperpathia (hyperalgesia): Increased reaction to a stimulus, especially a repetitive stimulus, as well as an increased threshold. Often painful.

Hypogeusia: Diminished sense of taste.

Hyposmia: Diminished sense of smell.

Jamais vu: The sensation of everything being strange and unfamiliar.

Jargon: Normal-sounding speech but made up of nonsense words.

Lethologica: Temporary inability to remember a proper noun or a name.

Moria: Euphoric and erotic behavior after a stroke or injury in the prefrontal cortex.

Neologisia: Use of word forms that do not exist.

Nystagmus: Involuntary, rapid, jerky movement of the eyeball.

Palinopia (palinopsia): Inappropriate persistence of a visual image after its removal.

Palinopsia (palinopia): Inappropriate persistence of a visual image after its removal.

Parablepsia: False vision such as a hallucination or illusion.

Paracusia: Abnormal hearing.

Paraesthesia: Tingling sensation on the skin.

Parageusia (ageusia, ageustia): Abnormality of the sense of taste.

Paragraphia: Miswriting when responding to a spoken word or number.

Parakinesia (akinesia, dyskinesia): Extreme reluctance to perform elementary motor activities. A form of apraxia.

Paralalia: Abnormal speech sounds.

Paralexia: Transposition of words or syllables.

Paramnesia: Abnormal memory of the meaning of words. Also used synonymously with the term *déjà vu*, meaning to have the illusory experience that something was previously experienced but is actually being experienced for the first time.

Paraphasia: Misuse of words, especially while talking.

Parapnasia: Incorrect word combinations.

Parasomia: Perversion of the sense of smell, especially the subjective perception of nonexistent odors.

Paresis: Partial or incomplete paralysis.

Perseveration: Inappropriate repetition of an action or behavior.

Prosopagnosia: Inability to recognize faces.

Protanopia: Color blindness in which red and green are confused.

Simultanagnosia: Inability to comprehend more than one element of a visual scene simultaneously or to integrate the parts into a whole.

Somesthesia: Disorder of sensation of touch, pain, temperature, limb position, or body sense.

Strabismus: Imperfect eye gaze coordination, such as cross-eyed or wall-eyed.

Synesthesia: An inappropriate sensory perception, such as perceiving a color in response to a particular odor.

Topagnosis: Inability to localize the site of tactile stimulation.

Topographagnosia: Inability to orient to an abstract spatial representation such as a map.

Tritanopia (acyanopsia): Color blindness in the blue region of the spectrum.

Verbal dysdecorum: Inability to self-monitor the appropriateness of speech in social settings.

Verbigeration: Inappropriate repetition of the last word spoken.

Witzelsucht: Inappropriate joking or factitious behavior after a stroke or injury in the prefrontal cortex.

Name	Functions
I. Olfactory	**Sensory**: Smell (olfaction).
II. Optic	**Sensory**: Vision (entire visual output of the eye).
III. Oculomotor	**Motor**: Innervation of all eye-movement muscles except the lateral rectus and superior oblique. Parasympathetic: Innervation of the iris and lens of the eye.
IV. Trochlear	**Motor**: Innervation of the superior oblique eye-movement muscle.
V. Trigeminal	**Motor**: Innervation of the muscles of mastication. **Sensory**: Facial touch, temperature, and pain including tooth pulp sensation, cornea, and extraocular structures.
VI. Abducens	**Motor**: Innervation of the lateral rectus eye-movement muscle.
VII. Facial	**Motor**: Innerevation of all face muscles except those for mastication. **Sensory**: Taste and sensation from anterior two-thirds of the tongue. Parasympathetic: Innervation of the lacrimal and salivary glands.
VIII. Vestibulocochlear (Auditory and Vestibular)	**Sensory**: Hearing and the vestibular-based sense of motion. At the brainstem level this is a combination of two sensory nerves, the auditory and vestibular.
IX. Glossopharyngeal	**Motor**: Innervation of the pharyngeal musculature. **Sensory**: Taste and sensation from posterior third of the tongue and sensation from the pharynx. Parasympathetic: Innervation of the parotid gland.
X. Vagus	**Motor**: Innervation of larynx, pharynx, and soft palate. **Sensory**: Visceral sensation from abdominal and thoracic organs, larynx, and pharynx; taste from posterior tongue and pharynx. Input from circulating stress-related hormones and immune system factors. Parasympathetic: Innervation of cardiovascular system, pulmonary system, and gastrointestinal system.
XI. Spinal accessory	**Motor**: Innervation of two major neck muscles, the trapezius and the sternocleidomastoid.
XII. Hypoglossal	**Motor**: Innervation of the tongue.

Action potential: The electrical signal that propagates along an axon.

Alpha motor neuron: The primary output neuron from the spinal cord to muscles.

Anterograde amnesia: The inability to form new declarative memories.

Axon hillock: The point on a soma where an axon originates.

Behaviorism: The theoretical concept that all brain function can be explained in terms of inputs and outputs only.

Binding problem: The question of how parallel processing properly associates the various parameters of a stimulus.

Bouton: A presynaptic swelling at the end of an axon branch.

Central pattern generator: A spinal cord circuit that coordinates complex patterns of muscle movement.

Cerebrospinal fluid (CSF): The specialized aqueous environment that nourishes and cushions brain tissue.

Cerebrum: Synonym for the cerebral cortex.

Channelopathy: A disease caused by mutated ion channels in neuronal membranes.

Choroid plexus: Specialized cells that produce cerebrospinal fluid.

Cognitive neuroscience: The theoretical formulation that internal correlates of meaning intervene in the brain between inputs and outputs.

Compulsion: An irrational repetitive behavior.

Computed tomography: A technique for reconstructing the three-dimensional representation of a structure from two-dimensional slices.

Concentration gradient: A difference of ionic concentration between the inside and outside of a neuron.

Cortical column: Neurons in a narrow cylinder of cortex perpendicular to its surface.

Critical period: A limited time early in postnatal development when a sensory modality experiences strong plasticity.

Cytoarchitectonics: A technique of classifying cortical regions by the fine details of neuronal distributions.

Declarative memory: Memory available to consciousness and able to be stated.

Decussation: Crossing of nerves from one side of the body to the hemisphere on the opposite side.

Dendrite: An extension from the soma that receives synaptic inputs.

Depolarization: A decrease in the voltage gradient across a neuronal membrane.

Dualism: The theory that there is a fundamental difference between physical and mental activities.

Electrical synapse: A synapse that allows direct flow of electrical current from the presynaptic to the postsynaptic side.

Electroencephalography (EEG): A technique for recording overall electrical activity of the brain.

Emotion: An automatic, autonomic response to a stimulus.

Episodic memory: Memory of a concept or idea that is embedded in a recollection of where or when it was learned.

Excitatory postsynaptic potential (EPSP): Postsynaptic depolarization that contributes to causing an action potential.

Feeling: The cognitive result of emotions.

Functional magnetic resonance imaging: A technique for measuring recently active areas of the brain.

Ganglion: A localized region of neuronal cell bodies outside of the spinal cord.

Glial cell: A type of cell that provides metabolic support and insulation for neurons.

G-protein: A second-messenger molecule inside a neuron.

Gray matter: A region of the brain predominated by neuronal cell bodies.

Gyrus (plural-gyri): A mountainlike expansion of the cerebral cortex.

Hair cell: A specialized, cilia-bearing cell of the cochlea that transduces sound vibrations.

Homunculus: The systematic representation of the body in the somatosensory cortex.

Hydrocephalus: A pathological enlargement of the ventricles.

Hyperpolarization: An increase in the voltage gradient across a neuronal membrane.

Implicit memory: Memory not available to consciousness, usually concerned with motor behaviors.

Inhibitory postsynaptic potential (IPSP): Postsynaptic hyperpolarization that inhibits the firing of an action potential.

Intelligence quotient (IQ): A purported measure of general intelligence.

Interneuron: A short-axon neuron that communicates locally with other neurons.

Ionotrophic transmission: A postsynaptic event in which transmitter binding causes direct opening of an ion channel.

Long-term potentiation: A change in synaptic efficacy as a result of recent neuronal activity.

Magnetic resonance imaging: A technique based on tissue density for imaging the brain.

Magnetoencephalography: A technique for recording overall electromagnetic activity of the brain.

Mechanoreceptor: A transducer for touch.

Memory trace: A hypothesized set of related neuronal interconnections purported to be related to a specific memory.

Metabotropic transmission: A postsynaptic event in which binding of transmitter causes the indirect opening of an ion channel via a second-messenger molecule.

Microelectrode: A thin, pencil-like device with a metal conducting core used to record from individual neurons.

Micropipette: A thin, pencil-like device with a fluid conducting core used to record from individual neurons.

Mood: A diffuse emotional state with no obvious immediate stimulus.

Myelin sheath: The lipid wrapping around an axon that allows for fast conduction of action potentials.

Na+/K+ ATPase: A molecular pump that moves ions across membranes.

Nerve: A bundle of axons, such as the optic nerve.

Neuron: An individual nerve cell.

Nocioceptor: A transducer for noxious stimuli.

Node: A small region of bare axon that interrupts the myelin sheath.

Nuclear magnetic resonance (NMR): Original name for the magnetic resonance imaging technique.

Nucleus: A localized collection of related neurons.

Obsession: A persistent idea usually associated with fear or doubt.

Opsin: The protein portion of light-absorbing pigments in the photoreceptors.

Outer segment: The region of a photoreceptor in which photons are transduced.

Parallel processing: The simultaneous analysis of different aspects of a stimulus in different regions of the cortex.

Patch clamp: A technique for recording from a small region of a neuronal membrane.

Peptide neurotransmitter: A small polypeptide that acts as a synaptic transmitter.

Phoneme: The basic unit of spoken sound.

Pixel: A single information element in a two-dimensional image.

Plasticity: The ability of neurons to form new connections throughout life.

Positron emission tomography (PET): A technique used for observing recently active areas of the brain.

Postsynaptic: The side of a synapse that contains receptors that bind the synaptic transmitter.

Presynaptic: The side of a synapse from which the synaptic transmitter is released.

Priming: The use of an unnoticed stimulus to facilitate recall of a memory related to that stimulus.

Prosody: The tonal aspect of language.

Qualia (singular-quale): The subjective experience of a sensation, such as the redness of an object.

Receptive field: The region in sensory space that a neuron responds to.

Reductionism: The theory that physical activity in the brain is all that exists.

Reflex arc: The minimum reactive circuit in the spinal cord.

Refractory period: The minimum time possible between sequential action potentials.

Resting potential: The negative voltage inside a neuron when it is unstimulated.

Reticulum: A loose syncytium of neurons that have related functions.

Retinotopic map: The orderly projection of visual space onto a cortical region.

Retrograde amnesia: The inability to recall past memories.

Rod monochromacy: The condition of only seeing shades of gray, usually due to the absence of cone photoreceptors.

Semantic memory: Memory of a concept or idea, without recollection of where or when it was learned.

Semantics: The meaning of words.

Semipermeability: The property of a membrane to allow passage of some ion species but not others.

Saltatory conduction: The jumplike movement of an action potential along myelinated axons.

Sleep spindle: A burst of high-voltage activity characteristic of light sleep.

Soma: The cell body of a neuron.

Spike: Colloquial name for an action potential.

Spin: The quantum property of an atom that is the basis of the magnetic resonance imaging technique.

Spine: A postsynaptic point of contact that extends from a dendrite.

Stretch receptor: A specialized structure in a muscle that provides feedback about muscle contraction.

Stroop test: A test for demonstrating ambiguity between the form of a stimulus and its perceived meaning.

Sulcus (plural-sulci): A slitlike valley between gyri.

Synapse: A point of functional contact between neurons, typically of a bouton to a dendrite.

Synaptic cleft: The narrow space between the presynaptic and postsynaptic side of a synapse.

Synaptic transmitter: A molecular that communicates between the presynaptic and postsynaptic side of a synapse.

Synaptic vesicle: A small, baglike organelle that contains synaptic transmitter.

Syntax: The grammatical construction governing the normal use of words.

Threshold: The value of the membrane potential that must be reached in order to trigger an action potential.

Transduction: The transformation of a physical, sensory stimulus into an action potential response.

Tuning curve: The receptive field of a neuron that deals with auditory stimuli, expressed in frequency space.

Ventricle: The enclosed region within the brain containing cerebrospinal fluid.

Voltage gradient: A difference of electrical potential between the inside and outside of a neuron.

Voxel: A single information element in a three-dimensional image.

White matter: A region of the brain predominated by myelin-covered axons.

Working memory: A transient form of short-term memory that stores a small number of recent concepts.